AOSpine Masters Series

Pediatric Spinal Deformities

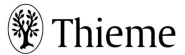

AOSpine Masters Series

Pediatric Spinal Deformities

Series Editor:

Luiz Roberto Vialle, MD, PhD
Professor of Orthopedics, School of Medicine
Cajuru University Hospital, Spine Unit
Medical Director, Human Tissue Bank
Catholic University of Parana State
Curitiba, Brazil

Guest Editors:

Sigurd H. Berven, MD
Professor in Residence
Chief of Spine Service
Department of Orthopaedic Surgery
University of California, San Francisco
San Francisco, California

Marinus de Kleuver, MD, PhD
Professor and Chairman
Department of Orthopedics
Radboud University Medical Center
Nijmegen, The Netherlands

With 173 figures

Thieme
New York • Stuttgart • Delhi • Rio de Janeiro

Thieme Medical Publishers, Inc.
333 Seventh Ave.
New York, NY 10001

Executive Editor: William Lamsback
Managing Editor: Sarah Landis
Director, Editorial Services: Mary Jo Casey
Editorial Assistant: Haley Paskalides
Production Editor: Barbara A. Chernow
International Production Director: Andreas Schabert
International Marketing Director: Fiona Henderson
International Sales Director: Louisa Turrell
Director of Sales, North America: Mike Roseman
Senior Vice President and Chief Operating Officer: Sarah Vanderbilt
President: Brian D. Scanlan
Compositor: Carol Pierson, Chernow Editorial Services, Inc.

Library of Congress Cataloging-in-Publication Data
Names: Vialle, Luiz Roberto, editor. | Berven, Sigurd H., editor. | Kleuver, Marinus de, editor. | AOSpine
    International (Firm)
Title: AOSpine masters series. V. 9, Pediatric spinal deformities / editors, Luiz Roberto Vialle, Sigurd H.
    Berven, Marinus de Kleuver.
Other titles: Pediatric spinal deformities
Description: New York : Thieme, [2018] | Includes bibliographical references and index.
Identifiers: LCCN 2017003720 (print) | LCCN 2017005643 (ebook) | ISBN 9781626234536 (alk. paper) | ISBN
    9781626234543 (ebook)
Subjects: | MESH: Scoliosis—surgery | Spondylolisthesis—surgery | Child | Adolescent
Classification: LCC RD771.S3 (print) | LCC RD771.S3 (ebook) | NLM WE 735 | DDC 616.7/3—dc23
LC record available at https://lccn.loc.gov/2017003720

Important note: Medicine is an ever-changing science undergoing continual development. Research and clinical experience are continually expanding our knowledge, in particular our knowledge of proper treatment and drug therapy. Insofar as this book mentions any dosage or application, readers may rest assured that the authors, editors, and publishers have made every effort to ensure that such references are in accordance with the **state of knowledge at the time of production of the book.**

Nevertheless, this does not involve, imply, or express any guarantee or responsibility on the part of the publishers in respect to any dosage instructions and forms of applications stated in the book. **Every user is requested to examine carefully** the manufacturers' leaflets accompanying each drug and to check, if necessary in consultation with a physician or specialist, whether the dosage schedules mentioned therein or the contraindications stated by the manufacturers differ from the statements made in the present book. Such examination is particularly important with drugs that are either rarely used or have been newly released on the market. Every dosage schedule or every form of application used is entirely at the user's own risk and responsibility. The authors and publishers request every user to report to the publishers any discrepancies or inaccuracies noticed. If errors in this work are found after publication, errata will be posted at www.thieme.com on the product description page.

Some of the product names, patents, and registered designs referred to in this book are in fact registered trademarks or proprietary names even though specific reference to this fact is not always made in the text. Therefore, the appearance of a name without designation as proprietary is not to be construed as a representation by the publisher that it is in the public domain.

Printed in China by Everbest Printing Ltd.
5 4 3 2 1
ISBN 978-1-62623-453-6

Also available as an e-book:
eISBN 978-1-62623-454-3

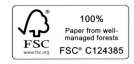
100%
Paper from well-managed forests
FSC® C124385

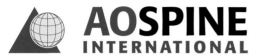

AOSpine Masters Series

Luiz Roberto Vialle, MD, PhD
Series Editor

Contents

Series Preface

Spine care is advancing at a rapid pace. The challenge for today's spine care professional is to quickly synthesize the best available evidence and expert opinion in the management of spine pathologies. The AOSpine Masters Series provides just that—each volume in the series delivers pathology-focused expert opinion on procedures, diagnosis, clinical wisdom, and pitfalls, and highlights today's top research papers.

To bring the value of its masters level educational courses and academic congresses to a wider audience, AOSpine has assembled internationally recognized spine pathology leaders to develop volumes in this Masters Series as a vehicle for sharing their experiences and expertise and providing links to the literature. Each volume focuses on a current compelling and sometimes controversial topic in spine care.

The unique and efficient format of the Masters Series volumes quickly focuses the attention of the reader on the core information critical to understanding the topic, while encouraging the reader to look further into the recommended literature.

Through this approach, AOSpine is advancing spine care worldwide.

Luiz Roberto Vialle, MD, PhD

Guest Editors' Preface

Deformity in the pediatric spine is common and clinically important. It encompasses a broad spectrum of pathologies, with significant variability in the age of onset of deformity, the natural history of deformity progression, and nonoperative and operative approaches to management of deformity. Knowledge of appropriate management, which is a priority for physicians, is evolving rapidly, and new classification systems, imaging techniques, and surgical approaches are contributing to changes in the evidence-based approach to optimal care. This book provides an overview of the best available knowledge regarding pediatric spinal deformity, encompassing conditions across a spectrum of ages and pathologies.

The first chapters focus on an overview of scoliosis, its classification and natural history, as well as nonoperative care. Subsequent chapters describe state-of-the-art surgical techniques for optimal management of early onset scoliosis and adolescent idiopathic scoliosis and present long-term outcomes of operative care, including indications and optimal strategies for safe revision surgery.

In the next part, the book focuses on kyphotic deformities of the pediatric spine, including spondylolisthesis and developmental kyphosis. Appropriate treatment of sagittal deformity in the pediatric patient is important to avoid disability in the adult. Many aspects of low- and high-grade spondylolisthesis are addressed, including classification and natural history, the relationship with idiopathic scolio-sis, and surgical treatment strategies. Chapter 14 provides an overview of other common kyphotic conditions affecting the pediatric spine, including congenital kyphosis, developmental kyphosis, and syndromic conditions that result in kyphotic deformity.

The final chapters address important health policy issues in pediatric spinal deformity. How can treatment of spine deformity be optimized in the developing world to include an effective infrastructure for complex spine surgery? In any setting, safety is the most important priority in making informed choices regarding appropriate care of the pediatric spine. While complications are inherent in complex spine reconstructions, strategies that may reduce the incidence of complications and improve the safety of patient care are important to review. The final chapter on outcome measures in pediatric deformity establishes metrics for quantifying the impact of deformity in the child and for measuring the result of the care and value we provide to society.

Our knowledge of pediatric deformity continues to evolve, and this book provides an up-to-date overview of our present understanding of optimal care. The authors and editors of this book provide the reader with information that should guide an evidence-based approach to care and will continue to guide changes to optimal care in the years to come.

Sigurd H. Berven, MD
Marinus de Kleuver, MD, PhD

Contributors

Kariman Abelin-Genevois, MD, PhD
Service de Chirurgie
Croix Rouge Française-CMCR des Massues
Lyon, France

Behrooz A. Akbarnia, MD
Clinical Professor
Department of Orthopaedic Surgery
University of California, San Diego
President and Founder
Growing Spine and San Diego Spine Foundations
San Diego, California

Ahmet Alanay, MD
Department of Orthopedics and Traumatology
Acibadem University School of Medicine
Acibadem Maslak Hospital
Maslak-Istanbul, Turkey

André Luís Fernandes Andújar, MD
Pediatric Orthopedic and Spine Surgeon
Chief of the Pediatric Orthopedic Surgery
    Department
Hospital Infantil Joana de Gusmão
Rodovia Gilson da Costa Xavier
Santo Antônio de Lisboa
Florianópolis, Brazil

Sigurd H. Berven, MD
Professor in Residence
Chief of Spine Service
Department of Orthopaedic Surgery
University of California, San Francisco
San Francisco, California

Oheneba Boachie-Adjei, MD, DSc
Professor Emeritus of Orthopaedic
    Surgery
Weill Medical College of Cornell
    University
Attending Orthopaedic Surgeon and Chief
    Emeritus
Scoliosis Service
Hospital for Special Surgery
Past President, Scoliosis Research Society
    (2008–2009)
Founder and President, FOCOS
New York, New York

Avery L. Buchholz, MD MPH
Complex Spine Fellow
Department of Neurological Surgery
University of Virginia
Charlottesville, Virginia

Kenneth M.C. Cheung, MBBS(UK), MD(HK), FRCS, FHKCOS, FHKAM(Orth)
Jessie Ho Professor in Spine Surgery
Head, Department of Orthopaedics and Traumatology
University of Hong Kong
Chief of Service (O&T)
Queen Mary Hospital
Hong Kong, SAR, China

Michael Dodds, MB, ChB
Departments of Traumatology, Pediatrics, Orthopedic Surgery
SickKids, Toronto
Toronto, Ontario, Canada

Sayf S.A. Faraj, BSc
PhD Candidate
Department of Orthopaedic Surgery
VU University Medical Center Amsterdam
Amsterdam, The Netherlands

Yazeed M. Gussous, MD
Associate Professor
Orthopedic Surgery
Ohio State University
Wexner Medical Center
Columbus, Ohio

Tsjitske M. Haanstra, PhD
Senior Researcher
Department of Orthopedics
Radboud University Medical Center
Nijmegen, The Netherlands

Manabu Ito, MD, PhD
Department of Spine and Spinal Cord Disorders
National Hospital Organization
Hokkaido Medical Center
Sapporo, Japan

Steven J. Kamper, PhD
Senior Research Fellow
George Institute for Global Health
University of Sydney
Camperdown, Australia

Sam Keshen, BSc
Department of Orthopaedics
Toronto Western Hospital
Toronto, Ontario, Canada

Marinus de Kleuver, MD, PhD
Professor and Chairman
Department of Orthopedics
Radboud University Medical Center
Nijmegen, The Netherlands

Faisal Konbaz, MD
Department of Orthopaedic Surgery
Johns Hopkins
Baltimore, Maryland

Kenny Kwan, BMBCh(Oxon), FRCSEd(Ortho), FHKCOS, FHKAM(Orthopaedic Surgery)
Clinical Assistant Professor and Honorary Associate Consultant
Department of Orthopaedics and Traumatology
Queen Mary Hospital
University of Hong Kong
Hong Kong, China

Michael LaBagnara, MD
Department of Neurosurgery
University of Virginia
Charlottesville, Virginia

Ekkaphol Larpumnuayphol, MD
Department of Orthopedic Surgery
Lerdsin General Hospital
Bangkok, Thailand

Lawrence G. Lenke, MD
Department of Orthopedic Surgery
Columbia University Medical School
Spine Hospital
New York–Presbyterian Hospital/Allen Hospital
New York, New York

Stephen Lewis, MD
Department of Orthopaedics
Toronto Western Hospital
University of Toronto
Hospital for Sick Children
Toronto, Ontario, Canada

Sergio Mendoza-Lattes, MD
Associate Professor
Department of Orthopaedic Surgery
Duke University Medical Center
Durham, North Carolina

Cristiano Magalhães Menezes
Hospital Ortopédico
Rua Prof. Otávio Coelho de Magalhães
Núcleo de Ortopedia e Traumatologia
Lourdes, France

Daniel J. Miller, MD
Chief Resident
Department of Orthopaedic Surgery
New York–Presbyterian Hospital
Columbia University Medical Center
New York, New York

Luis Eduardo Munhoz da Rocha
Hospital Infantil Pequeno Principe
Curitiba, Paraná, Puerto Rico

Joshua S. Murphy, MD
Pediatric Orthopaedic Surgeon
Children's Orthopaedics of Atlanta
Atlanta, Georgia

David W. Polly, Jr., MD
Professor
Orthopaedic Surgeon
Department of Orthopaedic Surgery
University of Minnesota
Minneapolis, Minnesota

Yong Qiu, MD
Spine Surgery
Drum Tower Hospital
Nanjing University Medical School
Nanjing, China

John C. Quinn, MD
Spine fellow
Department of Neurological Surgery
University of Virginia
Charlottesville, Virginia

Pierre Roussouly, MD
Service de Chirurgie
Croix Rouge Française-CMCR des Massues
Lyon, France

Zeeshan Mohammad Sardar
Advanced Spine Deformity Fellow
Spine Hospital
New York–Presbyterian Hospital/Allen Hospital
Columbia University
New York, New York

Christopher I. Shaffrey, MD
Professor of Neurological Surgery
Spine Division Director
University of Virginia School of Medicine
Charlottesville, Virginia

Justin S. Smith, MD PhD
Professor
Neurological Surgery
Co-Director
Neurosurgery Spine Division
Department of Neurological Surgery
University of Virginia
Charlottesville, Virginia

Durga R. Sure, MD
Department of Neurosurgery
University of Virginia
Charlottesville, Virginia

**Michael To, FRCSEd(Ortho), FHKCOS,
    FHKAM(Ortho)**
Clinical Associate Professor
Department of Orthopaedics and Traumatology
Queen Mary Hospital
University of Hong Kong
Hong Kong, China

Michael G. Vitale, MD, MPH
Ana Lucia Professor of Orthopedic Surgery
Columbia University Medical Center
Attending Physician
Associate Chief, Division of Pediatric
    Orthopedics
Chief, Pediatric Spine and Scoliosis Surgery
New York–Presbyterian Hospital
New York, New York

Irene Adorkor Wulff, MD
FOCOS Orthopaedic Hospital
Pantang–Accra
Ghana, West Africa

Katsuhisa Yamada, MD, PhD
Department of Orthopedic Surgery
Hokkaido University Graduate School of
    Medicine
Sapporo, Japan

Burt Yaszay, MD
Pediatric Orthopedic Surgeon
Rady Children's Hospital-San Diego
Assistant Clinical Professor
University of California–San Diego School of
    Medicine
San Diego, California

Caglar Yilgor, MD
Department of Orthopedics and Traumatology
Acibadem University School of Medicine
Istanbul, Turkey

1

Early-Onset Scoliosis: Classification and Natural History

Daniel J. Miller and Michael G. Vitale

Introduction

Although spinal deformity can occur across the spectrum of life, scoliosis in the young child presents unique challenges and treatment considerations given the ongoing growth of the spine and lungs. Early-onset scoliosis (EOS) describes the often severe, complex deformities of the spine and thorax, presenting in children younger than 10 years of age.[1] In fact, by virtue of differences in prevalence, comorbidities, and especially natural history, EOS is distinct from other forms of scoliosis both in terms of treatment strategies and outcomes.

The treatment of EOS remains a challenging and rapidly evolving area of pediatric spine care. A thorough understanding of the natural history of EOS is important in counseling families and treating patients. Treatment options must be continually and critically reassessed as the evidence base grows. This chapter discusses our understanding of the natural history of EOS, etiologies of EOS, and the recently developed Classification of Early-Onset Scoliosis (C-EOS).

Background

Early-onset scoliosis encompasses heterogeneous spinal disorders that are unified only in age and in the presence of spinal deformity.

The etiology of scoliosis in the EOS population varies widely and includes congenital scoliosis (i.e., congenital defects in vertebral formation and segmentation), structural scoliosis (i.e., scoliosis that results from fused ribs, chest wall anomalies, and congenital diaphragmatic hernia), scoliosis driven by neuromuscular diseases (e.g., cerebral palsy and muscular dystrophy), scoliosis associated with syndromes (e.g., neurofibromatosis, VACTERL [vertebral defects, anal atresia, cardiac defects, tracheoesophageal fistula, renal anomalies, and limb defects]), and scoliosis that arises in the absence of an identifiable cause (i.e., idiopathic scoliosis). Cognitive, functional, and medical involvement within this population varies from normal to severely impaired. Although the true prevalence of EOS remains poorly defined, EOS accounts for 10% of all pediatric scoliosis cases.[2]

Goals of management in EOS include regulating progression of spinal deformity, maximizing thoracic volume, and optimizing function and health-related quality of life while minimizing complications and negative effects of treatment.

Natural History

To understand and appreciate the effect of treatment options in EOS, one must understand the natural history of the disease. The heterogeneous population presents a dilemma when evaluating the effect of spinal deformity or treatment modalities on patients with EOS because existing comorbidities make it difficult to determine what symptoms and changes are attributable to the treatment, the scoliosis, or other medical issues. Comorbidities can be as significant in contributing to patient disability as the spinal deformity, and management by a multidisciplinary team is important for optimal care of patients with early-onset deformity.

Understanding the natural history of EOS is important in defining the incremental value of treatment. The literature on the natural history of untreated EOS is limited. Few patients with EOS remain untreated today, making the natural history of the disease difficult to determine. Studies are few in number, retrospective in nature, and limited by various forms of bias, such as a short follow-up period or a significant number of subjects lost to follow-up. Despite these problems, key studies have increased our understanding of EOS with respect to deformity progression, cardiopulmonary development, and clinical outcomes. This information serves as the foundation for current EOS treatment and ongoing research.

Thoracic Growth and Function

The three-dimensional growth of the thorax is of major importance in the treatment of patients with EOS, given the relationship between structure and function of the spine, thorax, chest wall, and lungs. A working knowledge of normal thoracic and spinal growth patterns affords a better appreciation of the pathological changes induced by early-onset spinal deformity.

Postnatal development of the lungs is characterized by substantial growth during the first 2 years of life. Pulmonary maturation then continues at a slower rate until age 8, at which time alveolar multiplication plateaus. Thoracic distortion secondary to extrinsic spinal or intrinsic chest wall deformity during these early periods can have a substantial deleterious influence on pulmonary development. Pulmo-

nary deficiency is particularly problematic for patients with neuromuscular scoliosis who may have limited ability to forcibly inhale or exhale secondary to muscular weakness.

An animal model of EOS in the rabbit demonstrates alveolar hypoplasia, decreased lung compliance, abnormal ventilation, and decreased pulmonary reserve.[3] Similar pathological and histological findings are reported in autopsies of patients with EOS.[4] Pulmonary function testing of patients with EOS demonstrates varying degrees of insufficiency secondary to pulmonary hypoplasia, decreased chest wall compliance, and muscular dysfunction.[5] Patients with severe EOS can also develop chronic cardiopulmonary issues such as pulmonary hypertension and subsequent cor pulmonale secondary to chronic vascular bed restriction and hypoxemia.[5]

Deformity Progression

Preventing curve progression remains a primary goal in the treatment of EOS. In the immature patient, the pattern of deformity progression is related primarily to the rate of spinal growth and the underlying etiology of disease. Accurate prediction of patterns of progression is important in guiding the timing of treatment and interventions.

Several authors have studied the growth of the normal spine. The T1–S1 spinal segment grows ~ 2 cm/year for the first 5 years of life followed by 1 cm/year from ages 5 to 10. Growth subsequently increases to ~ 1.8 cm/year until skeletal maturity.[6] These two periods of rapid spine growth (from birth to 5 years and from 10 years to maturity) correlate with periods of curve progression in both idiopathic and nonidiopathic scoliosis.[7] The following subsections briefly discuss the natural history of deformity progression with respect to each etiology of EOS based on the available literature.

Idiopathic Scoliosis

Idiopathic scoliosis occurs in otherwise healthy individuals without a discernible cause. Patients

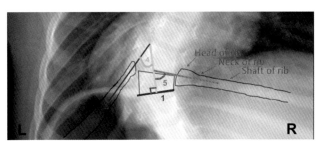

Fig. 1.1 The rib vertebra angle difference (RVAD), originally described by Mehta.[9]

Rib vertebral angle (RVA) = angle between apical vertebrae and its rib

1. Draw a line parallel to the bottom of the apical vertebrae (apical vertebra end plate).
2. Draw a line perpendicular to the line drawn in step 1.
3. Draw a line from the midpoint of the head of the convex rib to the midpoint of the nect of the convex rib to the line from step 2.
4. The resulting angle is the rib-vertebra angle for the convex side.
5. Repeat steps 3 and 4 for the concave side to calculate the RVA for the concave side.

Rib vertebra angle difference (RVAD) = RVA on the concave side minus the RVA on the convex side.

with idiopathic EOS typically follow a pattern of a progressive worsening or, in some cases, spontaneous resolution of curves.[8] Spontaneous resolution of deformity is a unique feature, as most other subtypes of EOS do not typically demonstrate deformity improvement. Reported rates of curve resolution vary widely in the literature between 20% and 80%.[8] Progressive curves tend to increase to a severe deformity given the large amount of growth potential within this patient population. Predicting whether idiopathic early-onset deformity will progress can be challenging, and it involves radiographic findings and a review of the pathoanatomy. The apical rib vertebral angle difference (RVAD) was described by Mehta[9] as a radiographic tool for identifying progressive curves in idiopathic EOS. The rib vertebral angle is formed between a perpendicular to the upper or lower border of the apical vertebra and a line crossing through the apical rib head and neck. The RVAD is the difference between the rib vertebral angle of the convex side and of the concave side of the curve at the apex (**Fig. 1.1**).

In a retrospective review of 138 patients with idiopathic EOS diagnosed before age 2, 80% of patients with progressive curves had an RVAD of > 20 degrees at initial presentation. In contrast, 80% of patients with resolving curves had an initial RVAD of < 20 degrees.[9] The utility of the RVAD in distinguishing between progressive and resolving curves in idiopathic EOS is supported by other authors,[8] though Corona et al[10] demonstrated variability in measurement of the RVAD.

Neuromuscular Early-Onset Scoliosis

Numerous factors contribute to spinal deformity in patients with neuromuscular disease, such as altered tone, intraspinal and congenital anomalies, impaired sensory feedback, and pelvic obliquity. The underlying etiology may be neuropathic or myopathic in nature. Neuropathic disorders can be further subdivided into upper motor neuron defects and lower motor neuron defects.

Although scoliosis patterns may vary within each neuromuscular disease, certain themes apply with respect to the prognosis of neuromuscular scoliosis among different subtypes. In general, a greater severity of illness is associated with a higher degree of spinal deformity. This principle is particularly evident in patients with spinal muscular atrophy and cerebral palsy, where the prevalence and degree of spinal deformity are intimately tied to disease severity and function. Poor trunk control and limited functional status are also associated with progressive spinal deformity.

Treatment of the young child with significant neuromuscular comorbidities presents challenges with regard to appropriate indications, technical approach, and outcomes given the frequency of complications in this patient population. Unfortunately, EOS can be a major contributor to the perturbations of health-related quality of life and to the natural history of patients with major neurologic comorbidities. At the same time, the risk of surgery and possible repeat surgeries must be carefully weighed and discussed with the patient's caregivers.

Congenital Scoliosis

Congenital scoliosis results from a failure of normal vertebral development during the 4th to 6th weeks of gestation. The incidence of congenital scoliosis is ~ 1 in 1,000 live births.[11] Anomalies are classified on the basis of failures of segmentation, formation, or both (mixed pattern).

Curve progression results from unbalanced growth on one side of the spine relative to the other and is influenced by type, location, distribution, and growth potential of vertebral anomalies.[11] The presence of fused ribs is associated with congenital scoliosis and increases the risk of deformity progression. Unilateral bony fusions (bars) act as growth tethers, whereas hemivertebra may act as an enlarging wedge. A wedge vertebra has bilateral pedicles, but hypoplasia occurs on one side of the vertebra. Abnormal bony fusion between adjacent vertebrae secondary to a defect of segmentation is termed block vertebra and is generally benign.[11,12]

A unilateral growth tether (bar) with a contralateral hemivertebra results in the highest rate of deformity progression (generally 5 to 10 degrees per year), followed by a unilateral bar, a hemivertebra, a wedge vertebra, and a block vertebra.[11,12] Multiple vertebral anomalies (mixed deformities) are less predictable, and the rate and severity of curve progression depends on the net asymmetry of growth potential and tethers on the spine.

Outcomes and Mortality

The cardiopulmonary consequences of severe EOS are an increased risk of substantial morbidity and mortality. Severe EOS that results in the inability of the thorax to support normal respiration or lung growth is termed thoracic insufficiency syndrome (TIS). Patients with TIS have a quality of life that is significantly impaired with regard to physical function and caregiver burden, one that is lower even than that of children afflicted with asthma, epilepsy, heart disease, or childhood cancer.[13]

Our best understanding of mortality in EOS comes from a long-term and much cited retrospective study by Pehrsson et al[14] of 115 women in Sweden. The authors report a 50% increase in mortality for patients with EOS from age 40 onward. Mortality was most significantly increased for the subset of patients with a diagnosis of scoliosis before the age of 3 and was not increased in patients with an onset of scoliosis after age 10. Patients with severe scoliosis (defined as curve > 70 degrees) had significantly increased mortality, whereas this was not true for patients with mild or moderate curves.

Classification

Classification systems are important for characterizing the nature of different conditions. They may help guide therapeutic interventions and may be used to predict the prognosis and outcomes of a disease state or treatment modality. Classification can also be important in research settings to facilitate communication and to ensure that different study populations are comparable.

The heterogeneous, skeletally immature patient population of EOS does not lend itself to existing classification systems for older patients with spinal deformity such as the Lenke classification of adolescent idiopathic scoliosis (AIS) or the Scoliosis Research Society–Schwab Adult Spinal Deformity Classification. Recognizing the importance of a reliable and valid classification system for EOS, members of the Growing Spine

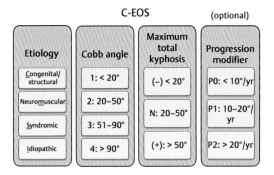

C-EOS   (optional)

Etiology	Cobb angle	Maximum total kyphosis	Progression modifier
Congenital/structural	1: < 20°	(–) < 20°	P0: < 10°/yr
Neuromuscular	2: 20–50°	N: 20–50°	P1: 10–20°/yr
Syndromic	3: 51–90°		
Idiopathic	4: > 90°	(+): > 50°	P2: > 20°/yr

Fig. 1.2 The Classification of Early-Onset Scoliosis (C-EOS) as described by Williams et al.[15]

Study Group (GSSG) and the Children's Spine Study Group (CSSG) collaborated to create the Classification of Early-Onset Scoliosis (C-EOS)[15] following a three-step model proposed by Audigé et al.[16] The C-EOS is applicable to all patients with EOS and is intended to be comprehensive, practical, prognostic, and directive.

The C-EOS (**Fig. 1.2**) has four components (age, etiology, major curve, and kyphosis) and an optional modifier (annual progression ratio, APR). Patient age (in years) at the time of classification represents a continuous age prefix. Etiology of spinal deformity is grouped into the following subsets: congenital or structural (including scoliosis related to chest wall abnormalities or iatrogenic in nature), neuromuscular (in which scoliosis is primarily attributable to a neuromuscular abnormality of tone), syndromic (in which the patient has a diagnosis of a syndrome that is associated with scoliosis that is not primarily related to congenital-structural or neuromuscular etiology), and idiopathic (in which there is no known cause of spinal deformity). The major curve angle is divided into groups based on the size of the major curve in the coronal plane in the position of most gravity: group 1, curve < 20 degrees; group 2, curve of 20 to 50 degrees; group 3, curve of 51 to 90 degrees; and group 4, curve > 90 degrees. Kyphosis is divided into the following three groups based on the magnitude of the maximal measurable kyphosis between any two levels in the sagittal plane: –, curve < 20 degrees; N, curve of 20 to 50 degrees; and +, curve > 50 degrees. An optional APR may be used to calculate the major curve progression over the course of two time points that are spaced a minimum of 6 months apart. This progression is scaled to the major curve progression per year as follows:

$$APR = [(\text{Major curve magnitude at time point 2}) - (\text{Major curve magnitude at time point 1})] / (\text{Time between t1 and t2 in years})$$

APR is divided into subsets, as follows: P1, < 10 degrees/year; P2, 10–20 degrees/year, and P3, > 20 degrees/year.

The C-EOS demonstrates substantial to excellent interobserver and intraobserver reliability as shown in both the original validation study by Williams et al[15] and in an independent evaluation by Cyr et al.[17] Case examples of the C-EOS are presented in **Figs. 1.3** and **1.4**.

Fig. 1.3 shows radiographs from a 4-year-old patient with spinal muscular atrophy (SMA), a form of neuromuscular scoliosis (M subtype). The magnitude of the major curve in coronal

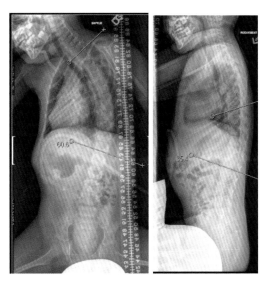

Fig. 1.3 Case example 1. Posteroanterior (PA) and lateral radiographs of a 4-year-old patient with spinal muscular atrophy (SMA). The magnitude of the major curve in the coronal plane is 60 degrees. The maximum regional kyphosis is 35 degrees. The major coronal curve was 35 degrees 6 months ago. The annual progression ratio = (60 degrees – 35 degrees/6 months) = (25 degrees/6 months) = (50 degrees/year). The final C-EOS classification is 4M3NP2.

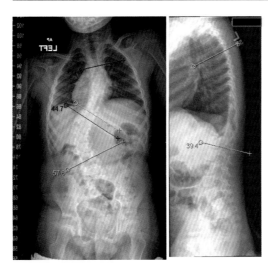

Fig. 1.4 Case example 2. PA and lateral radiographs of a 5-year-old patient with Angelman syndrome. The magnitude of the major curve in the coronal plane is 57 degrees. The maximum regional kyphosis is 39 degrees. The major coronal curve was 50 degrees 6 months ago. The annual progression ratio = (57 degrees – 50 degrees/6 months) = (7 degrees/6 months) = (14 degrees/year). The final C-EOS classification is 5S3NP1.

plane is 60 degrees (3 subtype). The maximum regional kyphosis measures 35 degrees (N subtype). The major curve in the coronal plane was 35 degrees 6 months ago, corresponding to an annual progression ratio of 50 degrees per year (P2 modifier). The final C-EOS classification for this patient is 4M3NP2.

Fig. 1.4 shows radiographs from a 5-year-old patient with syndromic scoliosis associated with Angelman syndrome (S subtype). The magnitude of the major curve in coronal plane is 57 degrees (3 subtype). The maximum regional kyphosis measures 39 degrees (N subtype). The major curve in the coronal plane was 50 degrees 6 months ago, corresponding to an annual progression ratio of 14 degrees per year (P1 modifier). The final C-EOS classification for this patient is 5S3NP1.

The C-EOS demonstrates significant prognostic value in predicting surgical complications in patients with EOS. In a review of 156 patients from the CSSG registry by Russo et al,[18] 105 patients (67%) had device compli-

cations, including 63 patients (40%) who had severe device complications requiring multiple, unplanned surgeries. More severe C-EOS categories (neuromuscular etiology, higher cobb class, and abnormal kyphosis) were associated with increased risks of device complications within this cohort. Park et al[19] demonstrated the ability to discriminate speed of proximal anchor failure between C-EOS subgroups in a retrospective review of 106 patients treated with the vertical expandable prosthetic titanium rib (VEPTR). The prognostic utility of the C-EOS may help provide surgeons and families with realistic goals and expectations from treatment.

We believe that the C-EOS will serve to standardize communication and facilitate future research efforts. With increased use, we are hopeful that it may have significant influence with respect to determining treatment and predicting outcomes in this difficult population.

Chapter Summary

Early-onset scoliosis describes the often severe, complex deformities of the spine and thorax that can affect young children as a result of a variety of medical conditions. Cognitive, functional, and medical involvement within this population varies from normal to severely impaired. Progressive spinal deformity can have severe deleterious effects on pulmonary development and function, leading to significant disability and early death. The C-EOS is a reliable and valid way to classify patients within this heterogeneous population.

Pearls

- EOS is defined as spinal deformity that is present before 10 years of age.
- The RVAD can help predict progressive and resolving curves in idiopathic EOS.
- Prognosis of neuromuscular scoliosis is associated with the patient's severity of illness and functional status.
- Curve progression in congenital scoliosis results from unbalanced growth of the spine and is influ-

enced by the type, location, distribution, and growth potential of vertebral anomalies.

◆ Severe and progressive spinal deformity can result in cardiopulmonary insufficiency and increase mortality.

◆ The C-EOS is a comprehensive classification system for patients with EOS that can help predict device complications.

◆ Failure to control curve progression during critical periods of pulmonary maturation.

◆ Underestimating the effect of thoracic insufficiency syndrome on quality of life.

◆ Failure to appreciate growth potential of certain congenital vertebral anomalies (e.g., unilateral bar with a contralateral hemivertebra).

References

Five Must-Read References

1. Skaggs DL, Guillaume T, El-Hawary R, Emans J, Mendelow M, Smith J. Early Onset Scoliosis Consensus Statement, SRS Growing Spine Committee, 2015. Spine Deform 2015;3:107

2. Riseborough EJ, Wynne-Davies R. A genetic survey of idiopathic scoliosis in Boston, Massachusetts. J Bone Joint Surg Am 1973;55:974–982

3. Olson JC, Takahashi A, Glotzbecker MP, Snyder BD. Extent of spine deformity predicts lung growth and function in rabbit model of early onset scoliosis. PLoS One 2015;10:e0136941

4. Davies G, Reid L. Effect of scoliosis on growth of alveoli and pulmonary arteries and on right ventricle. Arch Dis Child 1971;46:623–632

5. Yang S, Andras LM, Redding GJ, Skaggs DL. Early-onset scoliosis: a review of history, current treatment, and future directions. Pediatrics 2016;137

6. Dimeglio A, Canavese F. The growing spine: how spinal deformities influence normal spine and thoracic cage growth. Eur Spine J 2012;21:64–70

7. Duval-Beaupere G. [Maturation indices in the surveillance of scoliosis]. [Article in French]. Rev Chir Orthop Repar Appar Mot 1970;56:59–76

8. Fernandes P, Weinstein SL. Natural history of early onset scoliosis. J Bone Joint Surg Am 2007;89(Suppl 1):21–33

9. Mehta MH. The rib-vertebra angle in the early diagnosis between resolving and progressive infantile scoliosis. J Bone Joint Surg Br 1972;54:230–243

10. Corona J, Sanders JO, Luhmann SJ, Diab M, Vitale MG. Reliability of radiographic measures for infantile idiopathic scoliosis. J Bone Joint Surg Am 2012;94:e86

11. Hedequist D, Emans J. Congenital scoliosis: a review and update. J Pediatr Orthop 2007;27:106–116

12. McMaster MJ, Ohtsuka K. The natural history of congenital scoliosis. A study of two hundred and fifty-one patients. J Bone Joint Surg Am 1982;64:1128–1147

13. Vitale MG, Matsumoto H, Roye DP Jr, et al. Health-related quality of life in children with thoracic insufficiency syndrome. J Pediatr Orthop 2008;28:239–243

14. Pehrsson K, Larsson S, Oden A, Nachemson A. Long-term follow-up of patients with untreated scoliosis. A study of mortality, causes of death, and symptoms. Spine 1992;17:1091–1096

15. Williams BA, Matsumoto H, McCalla DJ, et al. Development and initial validation of the Classification of Early-Onset Scoliosis (C-EOS). J Bone Joint Surg Am 2014;96:1359–1367

16. Audigé L, Bhandari M, Hanson B, Kellam J. A concept for the validation of fracture classifications. J Orthop Trauma 2005;19:401–406

17. Cyr M, Hilaire TS, Pan Z, et al. Classification of early onset scoliosis has excellent interobserver and intraobserver reliability. J Pediatr Orthop 2015; PMID: 26600295

18. Russo C, Matsumoto H, Feinberg N, et al. Classification of early onset scoliosis predicts complications after initiation of growth friendly spine surgery. Presented at the American Academy of Orthopaedic Surgeons Annual Meeting, Orlando, FL, 2016

19. Park HY, Matsumoto H, Feinberg N, et al. The Classification for Early-onset Scoliosis (C-EOS) correlates with the speed of vertical expandable prosthetic titanium rib (VEPTR) proximal anchor failure. J Pediatr Orthop 2015;

2

Adolescent Idiopathic Scoliosis: Classification and Natural History

Zeeshan Mohammad Sardar and Lawrence G. Lenke

▨ Introduction

Children and adolescents between the ages of 10 and 18 can suffer from scoliosis caused by syndromic, congenital, neuromuscular, or neurologic conditions. However, if an etiology for the scoliosis is not found, it is classified as adolescent idiopathic scoliosis (AIS).[1] AIS is the most common type of spinal deformity in this population. Scoliosis is defined as a curvature of more than 10 degrees in the coronal plane. The normal alignment of the spine is straight in the coronal plane, whereas in the sagittal plane the thoracic kyphosis averages ~ 30 degrees and the lumbar lordosis averages ~ 55 degrees. AIS is much more common in females than in males and has a prevalence of about 1 to 3% for curves measuring 10 degrees or more.[1] AIS has a prevalence of ~ 0.1% for curves measuring at least 40 degrees.[2,3]

In general, management of AIS consists of observation, bracing, or surgery. For skeletally immature patients, observation is considered for curves less than 25 degrees, bracing is indicated for curves between 25 degrees and 40 to 45 degrees, and surgery is considered for curves greater than 40 to 45 degrees. Patients who are skeletally mature are typically not treated in a brace. In these patients, observation is indicated for curves up to 40 degrees and surgery is considered for curves greater than 45 to 50 degrees.

▨ Classification Systems

King Classification

In 1983, King et al[4] presented a classification system for selecting fusion levels in patients with idiopathic scoliosis. This classification system focuses on treating patients with posterior surgical fusion of the thoracic spine using Harrington rod instrumentation. Based on review of 405 patients, the authors identified five types of curves and recommended fusion levels.

Type I

An S-shaped curve in which both the thoracic and lumbar curves cross the midline. The lumbar curve has a higher Cobb angle than the thoracic curve by at least 3 degrees on standing X-rays, or the thoracic curve is more flexible on side-bending films. Both the thoracic and lumbar curves are fused in these patients. The lowest instrumented vertebra (LIV) is L4 or higher in all cases.

Type II

An S-shaped curve in which both the thoracic and lumbar curves cross the midline. However, the thoracic curve has a higher Cobb angle on standing X-rays, or the thoracic curve is less flexible on side-bending films.

King et al suggested either fusing both curves or performing a selective thoracic fusion. A type II curve of less than 80 degrees could safely undergo selective thoracic fusion if the LIV is stable.

Type III

Primarily a thoracic curve in which the lumbar curve does not cross the midline. Only the thoracic curve is fused in these patients.

Type IV

A long thoracic curve in which L5 is centered over the sacrum but L4 tilts into the long thoracic curve. The thoracic curve is fused in these patients.

Type V

A double thoracic curve with T1 tilted into the convexity of the upper curve. The upper curve is structural on side-bending films. King et al recommended fusing both thoracic curves in this type of curve.

Miscellaneous

Thoracic curves that do not fit the above five categories.

For type III, IV, and V curves, when performing a fusion, the stable vertebra is selected as the LIV. For patients undergoing thoracic fusion only, fusion distally beyond both the neutral and stable vertebra is not recommended.

Lenke Classification

The King classification system became widely used for the classification and treatment of idiopathic scoliosis even though it had poor to fair interobserver reliability.[5] However, the King classification was based solely on coronal radiographs and placed emphasis on thoracic curves. Lenke et al[6] recognized the need for a more reliable and comprehensive classification system that would consider the three-dimensional deformity encountered in idiopathic scoliosis, would have high inter- and intraobserver reliability, and would help in surgical decision making. They proposed a new, modular classification system in 2001 with three main components: curve type (1 through 6), lumbar spine modifier (A, B, C), and sagittal modifier (−, N, +). Thus, this new classification system aimed to define all types of curves while considering the deformity in multiple planes. The Lenke classification system is currently the most commonly used classification for AIS. Four radiographs are essential to classify curves using the Lenke classification: standing coronal and sagittal X-rays of the entire spine, as well as right and left side-bending views.

The coronal Cobb angles are measured on the upright coronal radiograph. Proximal thoracic (PT) curves are defined as those with the apex located between T3 and T5. Main thoracic (MT) curves have an apex between T6 and the T11-T12 intervertebral disk. The thoracolumbar (TL/L) curves have an apex between T12 and L1, whereas lumbar curves have an apex between L1-L2 and L4.

Side-bending radiographs are used to define structural curves. Curves ≥ 25 degrees on side-bending films are defined as structural curves. Additionally, the sagittal radiographs are used to assess structural curves. A PT curve is considered structural if the kyphosis from T2 to T5 measures ≥ 20 degrees. MT and TL/L curves are considered structural if the kyphosis from T10 to L2 measures ≥ 20 degrees. The major curve is the MT or TL/L with the larger Cobb angle on the standing PA radiograph. Thus, six main types of curves are defined:

Type 1: Main Thoracic

The MT curve is the only structural curve and is the major curve. This is also found to be the most common type of curve (40%).

Type 2: Double Thoracic

The MT curve is the major curve. However, the proximal thoracic curve is structural.

Type 3: Double Major

The MT curve is major, although both the MT and TL/L curves are structural.

Type 4: Triple major

The PT, MT, and TL/L curves are all structural. The major curve could be either the MT curve or the TL/L curve.

Type 5: Thoracolumbar/Lumbar Curve

The TL/L curve is the only structural curve and is the major curve.

Type 6: Thoracolumbar/Lumbar–Main Thoracic

The TL/L is major, although both the MT and TL/L curves are structural.

The lumbar modifier is assigned based on the position of the apical TL/L vertebra relative to the center sacral vertical line (CSVL):

Modifier A

The CSVL runs between the pedicles of the apical TL/L vertebra.

Modifier B

The CSVL touches the apical TL/L vertebra between the medial border of the concave pedicle and the lateral concave margin of the apical vertebral body.

Modifier C

The CSVL falls completely medial to the entire concave lateral aspect of the TL/L apical vertebral body.

Lastly, the sagittal modifier is assigned by measuring the thoracic kyphosis from T5 to T12. The normal thoracic kyphosis is between +10 degrees and +40 degrees with a mean of +30 degrees. Each curve can have one of the three sagittal modifiers:

- Minus (−): thoracic hypokyphosis when the kyphosis measures less than +10 degrees
- Normal (N): normal kyphosis between +10 degrees and +40 degrees

- Plus (+): thoracic hyperkyphosis when the kyphosis measure more than +40 degrees

A summary of the Lenke classification system is presented in (**Fig. 2.1**). Based on this classification, Lenke et al[6] recommended that the spinal fusion include only the major curve and the structural minor curves. At present, we recommend a posterior-only surgical instrumentation and fusion for AIS. A stepwise approach for selecting fusion levels based on the Lenke classification is as follows[2]:

Type 1: Main Thoracic

Instrumentation and fusion of the MT curve only. The upper instrumented level (UIV) is T3, T4, or T5. For lumbar modifiers A and B, the LIV is usually the most cephalad vertebra in the TL/L region at least intersected by the CSVL on the upright coronal radiograph. Selection of the LIV in curves with lumbar modifier C is more controversial. Lenke[2] recommends selecting the true stable vertebra at T11, T12, or L1 as the LIV in this case. However, in such a case it is important to under-correct the MT curve to allow harmonious transition into the lumbar spine. Selective thoracic fusion in Lenke 1C curves is more successful if the MT/TL-L ratios for Cobb magnitude, apical vertebral translation, and apical vertebral rotation are greater than 1.2. Additionally, the thoracolumbar kyphosis should be less than 10 degrees.[7]

Type 2: Double Thoracic

Instrumentation and fusion of both the PT and MT curves. The UIV is typically T2 or T3. The LIV is chosen in the same fashion as for type 1 curves. Special attention is paid to the clavicular/shoulder balance in these patients.

Type 3: Double Major

Instrumentation and fusion of both the MT and TL/L curves is recommended. The UIV is T3, T4, or T5. The LIV usually extends to L3 or L4. L3 is chosen as the LIV if the apex of the TL/L curve is at or cephalad to the L1-L2 disk, and the L3-L4 disk is neutral or closed on the convex

\multicolumn{5}{c}{**The Lenke classification for adolescent idiopathic scoliosis**}

Curve Type	Proximal Thoracic	Main Thoracic	Thoracolumbar/Lumbar	Description
1	Nonstructural	Structural*	Nonstructural	Main thoracic (MT)
2	Structural†	Structural*	Nonstructural	Double thoracic (DT)
3	Nonstructural	Structural*	Structural†	Double major (DM)
4	Structural†	Structural‡	Structural‡	Triple major (TM)
5	Nonstructural	Nonstructural	Structural*	Thoracolumbar/lumbar (TL/L)
6	Nonstructural	Structural†	Structural*	Thoracolumbar/lumbar main thoracic (TL/L-MT)

*Major curve: largest Cobb measurement, always structural; †minor curve: remaining structural curves; ‡type 4—MT or TL/L can be the major curve.

Structural criteria
(minor curves)

Proximal thoracic - Side-bending Cobb ≥ 25°
- T2-T5 kyphosis ≥ ⁺20°
Main thoracic - Side-bending Cobb ≥ 25°
- T10-L2 kyphosis ≥ ⁺20°
Thoracolumbar/lumbar - Side-bending Cobb ≥ 25°
- T10-L2 kyphosis ≥ ⁺20°

Location of apex
(Scoliosis Research
Society definition)

Curve	Apex
Thoracic	T2 to T11-12 disc
Thoracolumbar	T12-L1
Lumbar	L1-2 disc to L4

Modifiers

Lumbar Spine Modifier	Center Sacral Vertical Line to Lumbar Apex
A	Between pedicles
B	Touches apical bodies
C	Completely medial

\multicolumn{2}{c}{Thoracic Sagittal Profile T5-T12}

Modifier	Cobb Angle
– (Hypo)	< 10°
N (Normal)	10–40°
+ (Hyper)	> 40°

Curve type (1–6) + lumbar spine modifier (A, B, C) + thoracic sagittal modifier (–, N, +) =
curve classification (e.g., 1B+): _____

Fig. 2.1 A summary of the Lenke classification system criteria. (Reproduced with permission from Lenke LG, Betz RR, Harms J, et al. Adolescent idiopathic scoliosis: a new classification to determine extent of spinal arthrodesis. J Bone Joint Surg Am 2001;83:1169–1181.)

side of the TL/L curve. Otherwise, the L4 level is chosen as the LIV if the apex of the TL/L curve is at or caudad to L2, and the L3-L4 disk is convex or open on the convex side of the TL/L curve. A selective thoracic fusion may be considered in a type 3C pattern using the same criteria as the 1C pattern (**Fig. 2.2**).

Type 4: Triple Major

Instrumentation and fusion involves all three regions (PT, MT, TL/L). The UIV is chosen in a similar fashion to type 2 curves, whereas the LIV is chosen in a similar manner to type 3 curves.

Type 5: Thoracolumbar/Lumbar Curve

Instrumentation and fusion of only the TL/L curve is required. The UIV is usually one or two

levels above the upper end vertebra (UEV), whereas the LIV is the lower end vertebra (LEV) or one level below the LEV. Additionally, the factors used in selecting the LIV for type 3 curves should also be considered.

Type 6: Thoracolumbar/Lumbar–Main Thoracic)

Instrumentation and fusion of both the MT and TL/L curves is recommended. Selection of fusion levels is identical to that for type 3 curves.

Three-Dimensional Classification

Idiopathic scoliosis creates a spinal deformity in the coronal, sagittal, and the axial/rotatory planes. The Lenke classification system attempts to classify this multiplanar deformity by using

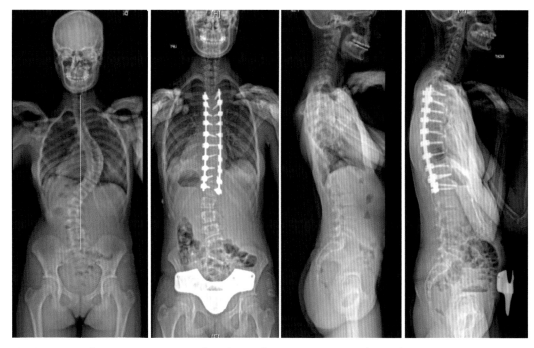

Fig. 2.2 Pre- and postoperative X-rays of a selective fusion in a patient with a Lenke 3C curve.

biplanar radiographs and is the most commonly used classification. However, attempts are ongoing to create a three-dimensional (3D) classification system for AIS. The Scoliosis Research Society's 3D Terminology Committee is actively working toward a 3D classification of AIS. One such 3D classification was proposed by Sangole et al[8] and Kadoury and Labelle.[9]

The objective of the classification by Sangole et al[8] was to analyze the presence of subgroups within the Lenke type 1 curves. They reviewed 172 patients with right thoracic Lenke type 1 curves. Biplanar radiographs were used to create a 3D reconstruction of the spine. These reconstructions were then used to compute the Cobb angle, thoracic kyphosis from T4 to T12, axial rotation of the apical vertebra, and the orientation of the plane of maximum curvature with respect to the sagittal plane. **Fig. 2.3** shows the 3D representation of a scoliotic spine. Each curve is identified by a triangle. The size of the triangle in the x-axis and y-axis represents the Cobb angle in the coronal plane and the kyphosis/lordosis in the sagittal plane, respectively. The z-axis represents the rotation of the vertebrae. This work showed that there

could be remarkable differences in the sagittal profiles of Lenke type 1 curves even when the curves had similar Cobb angles in the coronal plane. Additionally, the location of the apical vertebra in the coronal and sagittal planes may not always be the same.

Unfortunately, the use of 3D classification is currently limited as it involves complex calculations and requires the use of sophisticated computer software. Additionally, extensive research is still required to study the use of 3D classification in determining treatment strategies.

Natural History

The natural history of AIS varies considerably among patients and is dependent on age of onset, onset of menarche, curve pattern, curve magnitude, and skeletal maturity. These factors determine the progression of the curve in a patient with AIS. Lonstein and Carlson[10] reviewed 727 AIS patients with a curve magnitude from 5 to 29 degrees. They defined curve

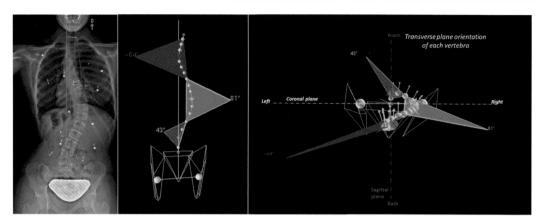

Fig. 2.3 Each curve is represented by a plane of maximum curvature *(triangle)* passing through the apex and the end vertebrae. In the transverse plane projection *(top view)*, the size of the triangles in the horizontal and vertical axes represent the Cobb angle in the coronal and the kyphosis/lordosis in the sagittal plane respectively. The vectors represent the rotation of the vertebrae. (Courtesy of Carl-Eric Aubin, chairman of the Scoliosis Research Society's 3D Terminology Committee.)

progression as an increase of at least 10 degrees in patients with curves less than 20 degrees, and as an increase of at least 5 degrees in patients with a curve of 20 degrees or more. Patients at high risk for progression were those with a curve measuring at least 20 degrees who had a Risser grade of 0 or 1 or those with a chronological age of 12 years or younger. Curve magnitude at presentation is considered to be the most important predictor of curve progression.[11] Thoracolumbar curves have the highest risk for developing lateral listhesis in adulthood,[12] most commonly at L3-L4.

The commonly noted negative outcomes associated with untreated AIS include curve progression, back pain, cardiopulmonary problems, and cosmetic and psychosocial concerns.[1] Patients with AIS may have more frequent and more severe back pain compared with the general population. However, that has not been shown to result in an increase in disability.[1]

Weinstein et al[13] reviewed the health and functional outcomes of patients with untreated idiopathic scoliosis at 50-year follow-up. They compared 117 untreated idiopathic scoliosis patients with 62 age- and sex-matched volunteers. Patients with a thoracic Cobb angle greater than 80 degrees were found to have an increased risk of shortness of breath, but that did not result in increased mortality. There was a higher incidence of back pain in the idiopathic scoliosis cohort; however, 68% of those patients reported little or only moderate back pain. Patients with untreated idiopathic scoliosis were found to be less satisfied with their body appearance compared with the control population.

Chapter Summary

Idiopathic scoliosis is the most common type of scoliosis in the adolescent population. It is a diagnosis of exclusion after other causes of the scoliosis have been ruled out. Scoliosis presents as a complex three-dimensional deformity in the coronal, sagittal, and axial planes. There are several classification systems for AIS. The Lenke classification is the most commonly used system at present. To classify a spine using the Lenke system, four radiographs are essential: standing coronal and sagittal X-rays, and right and left side-bending X-rays. This classification divides the curve into six patterns and further subclassifies them using the lumbar modifier and the sagittal modifier. Thus, the Lenke classification presents a reliable way of classifying AIS while also providing a treatment strategy. However, several other factors must be considered when determining levels for a fusion procedure, including the clinical appearance, the level of skeletal maturity, and the possibility of performing a selective fusion of the major curve.

The main shortcoming of the Lenke classification system is its reliance on biplanar radiographs for classifying curve types. Efforts are ongoing to establish a three-dimensional classification scheme for AIS. However, due to the complex nature of these schemes, they are currently not commonly used.

Pearls

- The Lenke Classification system is the most commonly used classification for AIS.
- The three main components of the Lenke classification are the curve type (1 to 6), Lumbar mod-

ifier (A, B, C), and the sagittal thoracic modifier (−, N, +).
- The Lenke classification offers a reliable system that facilitates communication among practitioners and guides surgical treatment.
- 3D classification systems are being developed but at present are not commonly utilized due to their complexity.

Pitfalls

- Be mindful of coronal side-bending and sagittal T2–T5 and T10–L2 measurements as they can change the curve classification and thus change the surgical plan.
- Evaluate UIV/LIV tilt during surgery to avoid "adding on" or decompensation.
- Pay careful attention to curves that are "rule breakers" such as a 1C curve that may require fusion of the nonstructural TL/L curve if the criteria for selective thoracic fusion are not met.

References

Five Must-Read References

1. Weinstein SL, Dolan LA, Cheng JC, Danielsson A, Morcuende JA. Adolescent idiopathic scoliosis. Lancet 2008;371:1527–1537
2. Lenke LG. The Lenke classification system of operative adolescent idiopathic scoliosis. Neurosurg Clin N Am 2007;18:199–206
3. Rose PS, Lenke LG. Classification of operative adolescent idiopathic scoliosis: treatment guidelines. Orthop Clin North Am 2007;38:521–529, vi
4. King HA, Moe JH, Bradford DS, Winter RB. The selection of fusion levels in thoracic idiopathic scoliosis. J Bone Joint Surg Am 1983;65:1302–1313
5. Richards BS, Sucato DJ, Konigsberg DE, Ouellet JA. Comparison of reliability between the Lenke and King classification systems for adolescent idiopathic scoliosis using radiographs that were not premeasured. Spine 2003;28:1148–1156, discussion 1156–1157
6. Lenke LG, Betz RR, Harms J, et al. Adolescent idiopathic scoliosis: a new classification to determine extent of spinal arthrodesis. J Bone Joint Surg Am 2001;83-A:1169–1181
7. Hoashi JS, Cahill PJ, Bennett JT, Samdani AF. Adolescent scoliosis classification and treatment. Neurosurg Clin N Am 2013;24:173–183
8. Sangole AP, Aubin CE, Labelle H, et al. Three-dimensional classification of thoracic scoliotic curves. Spine 2009;34:91–99
9. Kadoury S, Labelle H. Classification of three-dimensional thoracic deformities in adolescent idiopathic scoliosis from a multivariate analysis. Eur Spine J 2012;21:40–49
10. Lonstein JE, Carlson JM. The prediction of curve progression in untreated idiopathic scoliosis during growth. J Bone Joint Surg Am 1984;66:1061–1071
11. Tan KJ, Moe MM, Vaithinathan R, Wong HK. Curve progression in idiopathic scoliosis: follow-up study to skeletal maturity. Spine 2009;34:697–700
12. Agabegi SS, Kazemi N, Sturm PF, Mehlman CT. Natural history of adolescent idiopathic scoliosis in skeletally mature patients: a critical review. J Am Acad Orthop Surg 2015;23:714–723
13. Weinstein SL, Dolan LA, Spratt KF, Peterson KK, Spoonamore MJ, Ponseti IV. Health and function of patients with untreated idiopathic scoliosis: a 50-year natural history study. JAMA 2003;289:559–567

3

Preoperative Evaluation and Imaging Techniques in Adolescent Idiopathic Scoliosis

Kenny Kwan, Kenneth M.C. Cheung, and Michael To

Introduction

Optimal care for patients with adolescent idiopathic scoliosis (AIS) involves performing an appropriate preoperative clinical evaluation and requesting relevant imaging procedures for surgical planning. In the majority of patients, a proper history and a thorough physical examination, supplemented with plain standing radiographs of the whole spine, are all that is needed for diagnosis and treatment decision making. Additional evaluations may be needed for planning for surgery or bracing. The standing whole spine radiographs enable an appreciation of the two-dimensional deformities of the curvatures, whereas dynamic radiographs are important in determining curve flexibilities, which in turn influences the surgical approach, technique, and fusion levels. Computed tomography is occasionally needed to help delineate the bony anatomy and to exclude congenital causes. Magnetic resonance imaging is occasionally required to define the soft tissues and neural structures. This chapter discusses the preoperative clinical and radiological assessments in the planning of AIS surgery.

Preoperative Evaluation

History and Clinical Evaluation

Proper preoperative evaluation for patients with AIS should start by taking a history and performing a physical examination to exclude nonidiopathic neuromuscular, congenital, and syndromal causes. The history should address the age of onset and rate of progression, and the presence of symptoms and associated conditions. The age of onset defines if the scoliosis is considered early onset (before the age of 10 years) or adolescent onset. The main complaint is usually one of cosmesis; in other cases, the deformity has been discovered by a screening program or as an incidental finding in a routine clinical examination.[1,2] Thus, patients presenting with any symptoms related to the curvature should be thoroughly investigated. Night pain and back discomfort causing limitation in daily activities warrant more detailed investigations for underlying malignancy, chronic inflammatory disorders, and intraspinal abnormalities. The age of onset of puberty should be noted, which helps in assessing the skeletal

Table 3.1 Causes of scoliosis

Spinal Causes	Extraspinal Causes
Congenital	Pelvic obliquity
Neuromuscular	Leg length discrepancy
Syndromes (e.g., Marfan syndrome)	Sciatica
Idiopathic	Posture

maturity and the remaining growth potential; this age is easier to determine in girls, as the onset of menarche can usually be recalled, whereas in boys there is no clear clinical marker. The change of voice and the onset of growth spurt in boys may help to determine the skeletal maturity. The neurologic development of the child should also be properly evaluated to exclude possible underlying neuromuscular diseases. It is important to obtain a family history as well, as 30 to 50% of AIS patients have a positive family history.[3] The past medical history may provide a clue to the possible underlying diagnoses and is useful in determining fitness for surgery (**Table 3.1**).

The physical examination should confirm the diagnosis of AIS, evaluate the general fitness of the child, and assess the spinal malalignment and the flexibility of the scoliosis.

Adolescent idiopathic scoliosis is a diagnosis of exclusion, arrived at by ruling out other causes. Clinical features suggestive of syndromal diseases, skeletal dysplasia, and neuromuscular causes should not be overlooked. Café-au-lait skin lesions should alert the practitioner to the possibility of neurofibromatosis. Likewise, disproportionately long and slender limbs with long fingers and toes, joint laxity, and a high arched palate should raise the suspicion of Marfan's syndrome. The presence of sacral dimples, especially those associated with a tuft of hair, may suggest underlying spinal anomalies such as myelomeningocele and spina bifida. Patients with dwarfism, especially the ones with disproportionate short stature, should be assessed for skeletal dysplasia. A comprehensive neurologic examination is important to exclude spinal tumors, spinal cord anomalies (e.g., syringomyelia and tethered cord), and myopathies. Limb length should be measured to exclude secondary scoliosis from limb length discrepancy and pelvic obliquity. The presence of a joint contracture can affect the surgical decision making and needs to be carefully evaluated.

Although AIS is a three-dimensional deformity of the spinal column, its effects can extend to the whole truncal appearance and balance, which needs to be considered in the physical evaluation. With the child in the standing position, the front, back, and side should be properly assessed. Clinical determination of the structural curve(s) should be made, which, in our experience, is a useful adjunct to radiographic assessment. A proximal thoracic curve is indicated by a higher left shoulder and a trapezius line together with a prominent left scapula on forward bending (**Fig. 3.1**), whereas

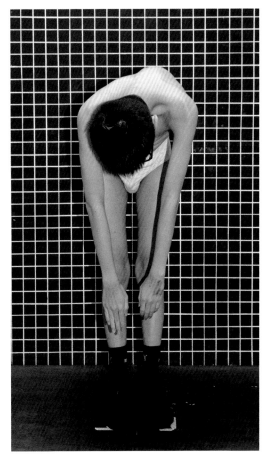

Fig. 3.1 A proximal thoracic curve is indicated by a prominent left scapula on forward bending.

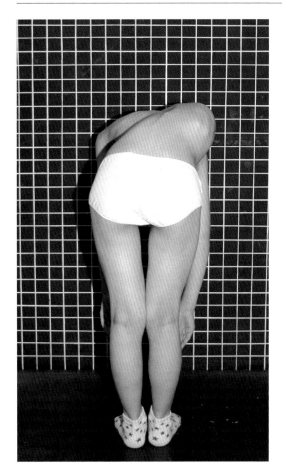

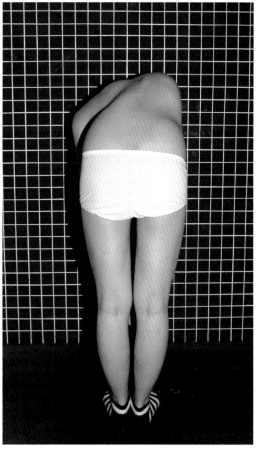

Fig. 3.2 A main thoracic curve is indicated by the presence of a rib hump on forward bending.

Fig. 3.3 A thoracolumbar curve is indicated by a thoracic and loin hump on forward bending.

a main thoracic curve is indicated by the presence of a rib hump (**Fig. 3.2**), and a lumbar curve, by a loin hump (**Fig. 3.3**). Rotational profile changes are best seen with the patient in the 90-degree-forward bending position and with the observer viewing from the back. In addition, with the patient in this position, have the patient actively bend to the left and right, which provides the examiner with a good sense of the amount of rotational correction of the curvature with coronal correction of the deformity (**Fig. 3.4**).

Listing, which represents the lateral translation of the head away from the midline, should be documented. It can be assessed by using a plumb line hanging down from C7 and by quantifying the lateral translation of the C7 relative to the gluteal cleft. Truncal shift refers to

the lateral translation of the rib cage in relation to the pelvis. Such assessment is particularly important in patients who have full head compensation with the head and neck back to the midline. Listing alone does not completely reflect the severity of the spinal deformity.

Proper recognition of the preoperative unleveled shoulders for the consideration of proximal thoracic (PT) curve fusion can help to prevent postoperative shoulder imbalance. In our experience, the preoperative left-elevated shoulder often necessitates the fusion of PT curve because sole correction of the right main thoracic (MT) curve can further elevate the left shoulder, whereas the preoperative right-elevated shoulder suggests that the PT curve fusion may not be required because the left shoulder elevation from the MT curve

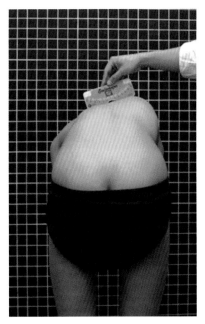
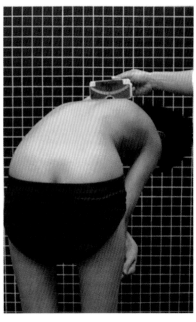

a   b

Fig. 3.4 Active side bending with the patient in the forward bent position can help to assess the amount of rotational correction and the flexibility of the curvature. Bending to the left **(a)** leads to an increase in the size of the hump, whereas right bending into the curve **(b)** results in a reduction in the curve and the size of the hump.

correction may be able to compensate the pre-existing right-elevated shoulder.

Neck Balance Evaluation

When evaluating the shoulder height in AIS patients, surgeons should not ignore the neck balance, especially in Lenke type 2 (double thoracic curve pattern) patients. In these patients, the T1 tilts to the right side due to the left proximal thoracic curve. The T1 can be considered as the "ground base" of the cervical spine. The T1 tilt is strongly associated with the neck tilt. Therefore, the neck also tilts to the right in these patients. It has been found that the neck tilt is distinct from shoulder imbalance.[4] Clinical neck tilting has poor correlation with clinical shoulder imbalance. Lenke type 2 patients with a preoperative right-elevated shoulder have good shoulder balance after partial fusion or non-fusion of the PT curve. However, these patients complain of postoperative deteriorated neck tilting due to the increased T1 tilt result

from decompensation of the unfused PT curve (**Fig. 3.5**). Full fusion of the PT curve with the correction of T1 tilt may be helpful in preventing the deterioration of neck tilting in these patients (**Fig. 3.6**).

We also assess the shoulder imbalance and asymmetry in AIS patients by determining the following: (1) shoulder height (**Fig. 3.7**), (2) shoulder area index 1 (**Fig. 3.8**), (3) shoulder area index 2 (**Fig. 3.9**), (4) shoulder angle (**Fig. 3.10**), and (5) axilla angle (**Fig. 3.11**).[5] These parameters can serve to supplement the radiographic parameters in surgical decision making for AIS patients.

Sagittal balance in AIS should not be overlooked. Patients with AIS develop thoracic hypokyphosis as a result of the rotational deformity. Some may also have reduced lumbar lordosis. Further reduction of thoracic kyphosis after surgery may lead to adjacent-segment disease and compensatory decrease in lumbar lordosis, resulting in disk degeneration, back pain, and poor quality of life.[6,7]

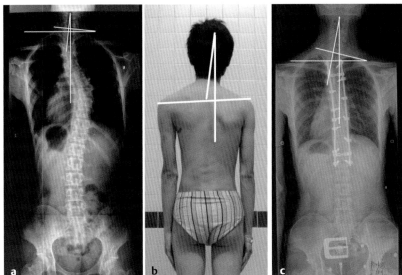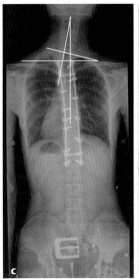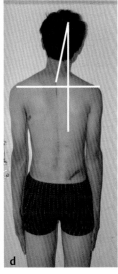

Fig. 3.5 (a,c) A 19-year-old man with preoperative radiographic right-elevated shoulder fused to T3. The neck tilt increased from **(b)** 4 degrees preopera-tively to **(d)** 11 degrees at the last follow-up. Although this patient had a leveled postoperative shoulder, the neck tilt deteriorated.

The findings regarding shoulder imbalance, listing, truncal asymmetry, abnormal thoracic, and lumbar deformity should correlate with the radiological assessment, so that all the information can be combined to address the correction of the scoliosis and the level of fusion. As the goal of AIS surgery is to restore the alignment of the spine and improve the cosmesis, the coronal and sagittal malalignment should be carefully assessed.

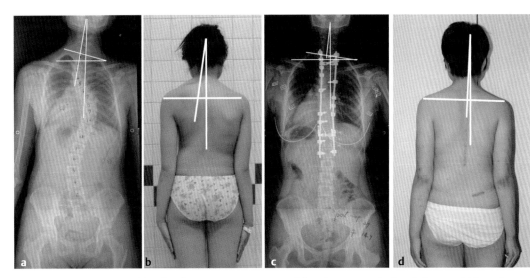

Fig. 3.6 (a,c) A 12-year-old girl with preoperative right-elevated shoulder fused to T1. The neck tilt was corrected from **(a)** 13 degrees preoperatively, to **(d)** 6 degrees at the last follow-up. This patient had both good neck balance and shoulder symmetry.

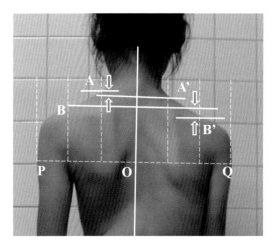

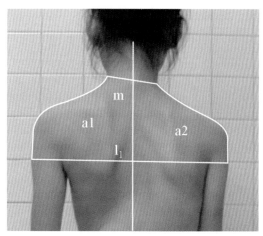

Fig. 3.7 Shoulder height (SH): The horizontal line through the higher axilla intersects the arms at *P (left)* and *Q (right)*, the plumb line through the midpoint of the neck intersects this horizontal line at *O*, and the trisection lines of *OP, OQ* intersect the shoulders at *A′, B′ (right)*. The difference between the heights of *A* and *A′* is defined as the inner shoulder height (SHi), and that between *B* and *B′* is defined as the outer shoulder height (SHo)

Fig. 3.8 Shoulder area index 1 (SAI1): The area surrounded by m, l_1, the superior margin of the shoulders and the outer margin of the upper arms, is divided by the plumb line through the midpoint of the neck into area *a1* and area *a2*; the ratio *a1/a2* is defined as SAI1. [m is the line connecting the two inflection points *(right and left)* between the shoulder and neck; l_1 is the horizontal line through the higher axilla.]

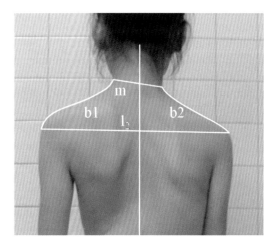

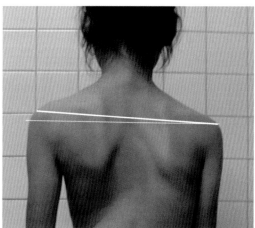

Fig. 3.9 Shoulder area index 2 (SAI2): The area surrounded by m, l_2, the superior margin of the shoulders, is divided by the plumb line through the midpoint of the neck into area *b1* and area *b2*; the ratio *b1/b2* is defined as SAI2. [m is the line connecting the two inflection points *(right and left)* between the shoulder and neck; l_2 is the horizontal line through the lower inflection point between the shoulder and the upper arm.]

Fig. 3.10 Shoulder angle: the angle between the horizontal line and the line through two inflection points of the shoulders and upper arms.

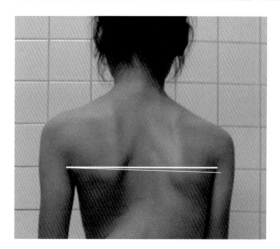

Fig. 3.11 Axilla angle: the angle between the horizontal line and the line through both axillae.

Other Preoperative Assessment and Preparation

Pulmonary function test is routinely used in some centers for preoperative assessment. According to the Delphi survey conducted by the AOSpine Knowledge Forum Deformity group, 50% of the experts considered pulmonary function tests as optimal care for AIS patients with Cobb angle curves between 40 and 90 degrees or for routine care scenarios.[8] Increasing coronal and sagittal plane deformities with a high thoracic scoliosis apex is associated with reduced forced vital capacity.[9] However, the degrees of scoliosis that were associated with a clinically relevant decrease in pulmonary function were much smaller. In a retrospective review of patients with severe scoliosis (Cobb angle ≥ 100 degrees), patients with severe restrictive pulmonary dysfunction [i.e., forced vital capacity (FVC) ratio ≤ 65%, forced expiratory volume at the end of the first second (FEV1) ratio ≤ 65%, and peak expiratory flow (PEF) ratio ≤ 65%.][10] had a higher incidence of postoperative pulmonary complications, and thoracoplasty was determined to be highly associated with such complications. The incidence of postoperative pulmonary complications increase significantly from 2.72% at FVC ratio ≥ 60% to 31.60% at FVC ratio < 40%.[11] We routinely arrange a postoperative intensive care unit placement for ventilator support for patients with severe restrictive pulmonary dysfunction.

Although AIS patients are usually not taking regular medications, drugs such as nonsteroidal anti-inflammatory drugs (NSAIDs) and oral contraceptives should be stopped before the surgery, as NSAIDs are known to increase blood loss and oral contraceptives can increase the risk of developing thromboembolism. Preoperative iron supplements and erythropoietin and preoperative autologous blood donation have been shown to reduce homologous blood transfusion to reduce the risk of disease transmission and adverse immunologic reaction. However, according to the Delphi survey, autologous blood donation and erythropoietin are used by only 37% and 17% of practitioners, respectively, as a means of blood conservation.[8] More recent reports find that there is a declining utilization rate of autologous blood donation,[12] and erythropoietin is not considered cost-effective. Other intraoperative measures have been adopted to reduce blood loss for scoliosis surgery, such as controlled hypotensive anesthesia, Cell Saver, and tranexamic acid.[13] We still favor the use of preoperative autologous blood donation to avoid allogeneic transfusion for the patients.

Psychological Evaluation and Preparation

Scoliosis surgery can be psychologically stressful to the patients as well as the families. Concerns about unsightly scars, pain, lack of social support, and adjustment of lifestyles after the surgery are not uncommon. Psychological stress can in turn affect significantly the postoperative pain control. To help relieve psychological stress, we recommend a detailed preoperative discussion, tour of the surgical units, and clinical psychologist evaluation to help better prepare patients before the surgery and to ameliorate their anxiety.

Imaging Techniques

Plain Radiographs

The standard preoperative radiographic assessment for AIS should include a standing postero-anterior (PA) and lateral whole spine radiographs or their equivalent, flexibility radiographs, and active side-bending radiographs.

The PA radiographs should be evaluated for any osseous anomaly to exclude congenital scoliosis and confirm the diagnosis of AIS. The type of curve can be classified accordingly, and the magnitude of each curve is measured by the Cobb angles. The presence of a structural proximal thoracic (PT) curve is diagnosed by the presence of a positive T1 tilt, elevation of the shoulder, and apical vertebral rotation (AVR). A positive T1 tilt is defined as the angle between the proximal end plate of T1 and the horizontal with the left proximal vertebral body directed upward and the right lower vertebral body directed downward (**Fig. 3.12**). Radiographic shoulder height (RSH) is used to evaluate the shoulder height imbalance with consideration of soft tissue above the shoulders (**Fig. 3.13**). AVR is assessed by the asymmetry of the pedicle shadow at the apex, according to the Nash and Moe method.

Apart from the structural PT curve, preoperative unleveled shoulder and neck tilt are important factors in considering whether the PT curve should be included in the fusion block.[14,15] However, it has been demonstrated that no radiographic parameter correlates perfectly with clinical shoulder symmetry.[5] In patients with elevated left shoulder, correction of the MT curve only may risk further elevation of the left shoulder postoperatively. Conversely, patients with elevated right shoulders will be compensated postoperatively after correction of the MT curve, although there is a risk of decompensation due to the more powerful instrumentation and correction of MT curves available today. Hence, the surgeon should take into account the flexibility of the curves as well as the clinical shoulder levels. The ultimate decision of whether the proximal thoracic curve should be instrumented, once it is diagnosed, is controversial and needs to be individualized for each patient, based on the clinical and radiological appearance.

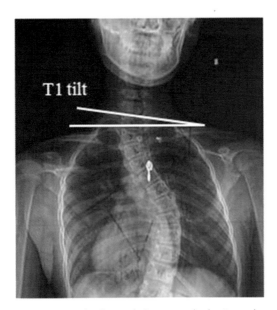

Fig. 3.12 T1 tilt: the angle between the horizontal line and the line through the upper end plate of T1. The value is positive if T1 tilts to the right and negative if T1 tilts to the left.

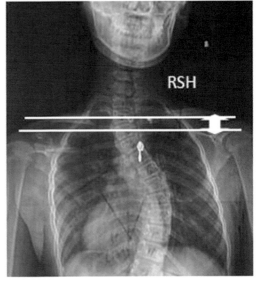

Fig. 3.13 Radiographic shoulder height (RSH): the difference in the soft tissue shadow directly superior to the acromioclavicular joint. The value is positive if the left is higher and negative if the right is higher.

Truncal balance assessment is an important radiological index in the standing PA radiographs. The magnitude and ratio of the MT-thoracolumbar/lumbar curves, and the thoracic and lumbar apical horizontal translation from the central sacral vertical line (CSVL) can be measured. In contrast with shoulder balance, radiographic truncal shift is significantly correlated with cosmetic truncal shift, with thoracic apical translation from the CSVL having the greatest correlation.[16]

Preoperative assessment of the lumbar deformity is important in determining the spinal balance and its relationship with the proximal curves. Pelvic obliquity needs to be taken into consideration, and limb length discrepancy needs to be corrected before obtaining the radiographs. The relationship of the apex of the lumbar curve to CSVL is classified into lumbar modifier A, B, and C types in the Lenke classification. When the CSVL falls medial to the entire concave lateral aspect of the thoracolumbar or lumbar apex (modifier C), the lumbar curve should be included in the arthrodesis.

On the lateral radiographs, measurements of the sagittal profile include thoracic kyphosis (TK), lumbar lordosis (LL), and the sagittal vertical axis (SVA). According to a prospective study by Horton et al,[17] the optimal patient positioning for a full-length lateral radiograph is with the hands on the clavicles and with the hips being visible. There is no consensus in the literature on the definition of a fixed Cobb measurement, but T2–T5, T5–T12, T10–L2 are commonly used because these measurements define structurality and form the sagittal thoracic modifier in the Lenke classification. However, regional kyphosis reliability is poor, particularly in the upper thoracic spine due to structural overlap of anatomic structures. Some have advocated a nonfixed TK measurement based on the individual sagittal shape of the spine. In the Lenke classification, a thoracic or thoracolumbar kyphosis in the minor curves, defined as 20 degrees or more, is considered structural, and the thoracic sagittal modifier defines T5–T12 as hypokyphotic if it is less than 10 degrees, normal if it is between 10 and 40 degrees, and hyperkyphotic if it is more than 40 degrees.

Flexibility Radiographs

Perhaps one of the most important preoperative radiographic assessments for AIS is determining the flexibility of the curves. An ideal dynamic radiograph should demonstrate the intrinsic stiffness of the curves preoperatively, enabling the surgeon to plan the type of osteotomy and anterior release if required to correct the curve, to select fusion levels, and to predict the postoperative outcome. A Delphi survey conducted by the AOSpine Knowledge Forum Deformity group on optimal surgical care for AIS found that there was no consensus as to which type of dynamic radiograph was optimal in assessing flexibility.[8] Some of the methods of assessment include fulcrum side-bending over a bolster, traction, prone push, and supine side-bending radiographs.

The Lenke classification defines structurality of the minor coronal curves based on a supine side-bending radiograph. If there is a residual coronal Cobb angle of 25 degrees or more on side-bending radiographs, this is considered structural and should be included in the fusion block. However, as the structural definition is arbitrary, surgeons attempting to save levels may not strictly follow these guidelines, as demonstrated by the proportion of "rule breakers" in Lenke type 3, 4, and 6 curves.[18]

However, the main disadvantage of a supine side-bending radiograph is that it requires active cooperation and effort by the patient, so the degree of curve flexibility is patient-dependent. To overcome this disadvantage, Cheung and Luk[19] described the fulcrum bending radiograph (FBR), which uses a bolster placed under the rib corresponding to the apex of the thoracic curve (**Fig. 3.14**). This passive and reproducible bending force accurately predicts the postoperative correction with pedicle screw fixation systems.[19–21] In view of the ability of the FBR to predict postoperative correction, a method was proposed to use the FBR to determine fusion levels in selective thoracic curves.[22]

An active lumbosacral (LS) bending radiograph should be obtained in the presence of a structural lumbar or thoracolumbar curve. The main purpose is to determine the lowest

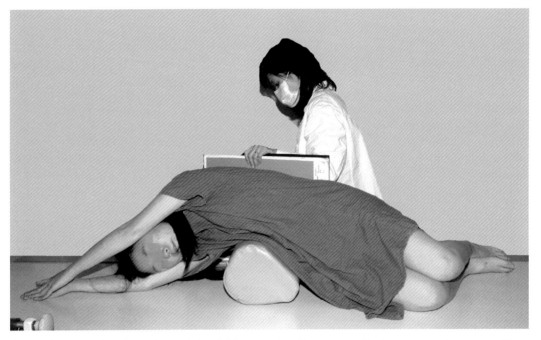

Fig. 3.14 Fulcrum bending radiograph (FBR): The patient is positioned on the lateral decubitus position. A padded cylinder (fulcrum) of appropriate size is placed on the side of the curve at the level of the rib corresponding to the apex of the curve. The fulcrum should be positioned to allow the shoulder and the pelvis to be lifted off the table.

instrumented vertebra (LIV) in the context of a lumbar curve fusion. On an active LS bend, if the vertebra caudal to the end vertebra is square compared with the pelvis and the disk space between the two can open, then the end vertebra can be chosen as the LIV. However, in the case of fixed L5 obliquity, fusion should be extended into the sacrum.

Role of Traction in the Preoperative Period and in the Operating Room

In routine cases of AIS where the curve pattern is typical and the curve is not rigid, the AOSpine Delphi survey found that performing preoperative traction was not considered part of optimal care (98%).[8]

The published evidence concerning intraoperative traction in AIS surgery applies to large rigid curves of over 100 degrees, and its use should not be considered routine.[23,24]

Assessment of Skeletal Maturity

The pelvis is normally included in a whole spine radiograph, and the degree of iliac apophysis development, known as the Risser sign, is the most frequently used indirect measure of skeletal maturity. Joseph C. Risser first described the state of ossification of the iliac apophysis, which was proportional to the state of a patient's spinal skeletal maturity. Two different versions of the Risser system are in use; the United States Risser staging system divides the excursion of the apophysis into quarters of the iliac crest beginning anterolaterally and progressing posteromedially, whereas the French Risser staging system divides the excursion of the apophysis into thirds.[25] However, there is a high frequency of anomalous apophysis development and disagreement between the anteroposterior (AP) and PA film of the pelvis. Hence, this should not be the single measure of skeletal maturity in clinical practice.

A radiograph of the hand and wrist should be taken on a yearly or more frequent basis to acquire more information in determining the stage of maturity. Estimation of the skeletal age is based on the appearance of the epiphyses of the phalanges from the earliest stages of ossification until fusion with the diaphysis, as described by Greulich and Pyle.[26] Furthermore, Sanders et al[27] showed that according to the Tanner and Whitehouse (TW3) digital skeletal age, "capping" of the finger epiphysis maturation is closely related to the peak height velocity.

However, both the Risser sign and peak height velocity according to digital epiphyseal closure have limitations in assessing skeletal maturity and do not correspond well with cessation of growth and risk of curve progression. In response to this, the distal radius and ulnar (DRU) classification was created and reported by Luk et al.[28] This classification, which included 11 radius grades (R1 to R11) and nine ulna grades (U1 to U9), was found to determine accurately the peak height velocity (R7 and U5) and cessation of growth (R10 and U9). Menarche occurs one to two stages after the peak height velocity. This strong association can help clinicians decide between bracing and surgery.

Computed Tomography (CT)

In most routine AIS cases, a preoperative CT of the spine is not necessary. It exposes the child to unnecessary radiation without clear benefits. However, there may be special circumstances where additional understanding of the spinal anatomy and deformity may help with preoperative planning. In a neglected or severe long-standing AIS patient where the anatomy is altered, visualization of the pedicles on plain radiographs is not clear or possible, and CT images can help with preoperative planning. If computer-assisted navigation is planned for the insertion of pedicle screws, a preoperative CT scan may also be needed to enable intraoperative matching. There are a small number of retrospective studies that report a more accurate screw placement, but not increased safety (fewer complications of pedicle screws, fewer re-interventions) using computer-assisted navigation.

Magnetic Resonance Imaging (MRI)

There was no consensus from the Delphi survey on obtaining routine preoperative full-spine MRI for AIS patients, but Winter et al[29] found that the incidence of intraspinal abnormality in routine AIS cases was low, and routine MRI was probably not indicated. Nonetheless, an MRI is indicated in the presence of any of the following findings: an atypical curve pattern (a left-sided short sharp thoracic curve, a right-sided thoracolumbar curve), an abnormal neurologic examination of the lower limb or foot deformity, absent or asymmetrical abdominal reflex, skin stigmata of neurofibromatosis, or occult spinal dysraphism.

The purpose of a complete spinal axis MRI is to detect any undiagnosed intraspinal pathology, which can be correctible causes of scoliosis, and to evaluate conditions that should be treated before surgical correction. Spinal dysraphic anomalies include tethered cord, syringohydromyelia, Chiari malformations, diastematomyelia, meningo- or myelomeningocele, and intraspinal lipoma. Occasionally, it is possible to detect vertebral or intraspinal tumors that can predispose to spinal deformity. Osteoid osteoma and osteoblastoma are the commonest primary vertebral tumors associated with scoliosis, and intraspinal tumors, which can be intramedullary (e.g., astrocytoma) or extramedullary (e.g., neurofibroma, meningioma, lipoma, dermoid cyst), can be encountered.

▥ Chapter Summary

The aims of preoperative imaging in AIS are to assess the structure and flexibility of the curves, determine shoulder and coronal truncal balance, and appreciate the sagittal profile, so as to plan the best operative strategy. Additional imaging is sometimes required to exclude undetected pathologies that may render the scoliosis secondary, or to aid operative planning. Although an important goal of AIS surgery is correction of certain radiographic parameters, it is increasingly recognized that the success of surgical correction is determined by the cosmetic result and patient satisfaction. The surgeon must therefore carefully consider the clinical evaluation, and correlate the findings with radiological assessment to accomplish a balance and symmetrical outcome postoperatively.

Pearls

◆ Thorough history and physical examination are required to assess the etiology, structure, and flexibility of the curve.
◆ Standing whole spine posteroanterior and lateral radiographs including the hips and some form of dynamic radiographs are obtained for all AIS patients.

◆ Use of preoperative and intraoperative traction is not recommended in routine case scenarios.
◆ MRI should be obtained in atypical curves or the presence of abnormal findings on neurologic examination to exclude underlying intraspinal abnormalities.

Pitfalls

◆ Failure to examine the patients clinically and over-reliance on the radiological index can result in cosmetically displeasing results.
◆ Selection of fusion levels without taking into consideration of curve flexibility will result in over- or undercorrection.

Acknowledgment

We wish to acknowledge Qiu Yong for contributing to the section on shoulder balance.

References
Five Must-Read References

1. Lee CF, Fong DY, Cheung KM, et al. A new risk classification rule for curve progression in adolescent idiopathic scoliosis. Spine J 2012;12:989–995
2. Fong DY, Cheung KM, Wong YW, et al. A population-based cohort study of 394,401 children followed for 10 years exhibits sustained effectiveness of scoliosis screening. Spine J 2015;15:825–833
3. Grauers A, Danielsson A, Karlsson M, Ohlin A, Gerdhem P. Family history and its association to curve size and treatment in 1,463 patients with idiopathic scoliosis. Eur Spine J 2013;22:2421–2426
4. Kwan MK, Wong KA, Lee CK, Chan CY. Is neck tilt and shoulder imbalance the same phenomenon? A prospective analysis of 89 adolescent idiopathic scoliosis patients (Lenke type 1 and 2). Eur Spine J 2016; 25:401–408
5. Qiu XS, Ma WW, Li WG, et al. Discrepancy between radiographic shoulder balance and cosmetic shoulder balance in adolescent idiopathic scoliosis patients with double thoracic curve. Eur Spine J 2009;18: 45–51
6. Hwang SW, Samdani AF, Tantorski M, et al. Cervical sagittal plane decompensation after surgery for adolescent idiopathic scoliosis: an effect imparted by postoperative thoracic hypokyphosis. J Neurosurg Spine 2011;15:491–496

7. Ilharreborde B, Morel E, Mazda K, Dekutoski MB. Adjacent segment disease after instrumented fusion for idiopathic scoliosis: review of current trends and controversies. J Spinal Disord Tech 2009;22:530–539
8. de Kleuver M, Lewis SJ, Germscheid NM, et al. Optimal surgical care for adolescent idiopathic scoliosis: an international consensus. Eur Spine J 2014;23: 2603–2618
9. Dreimann M, Hoffmann M, Kossow K, Hitzl W, Meier O, Koller H. Scoliosis and chest cage deformity measures predicting impairments in pulmonary function: a cross-sectional study of 492 patients with scoliosis to improve the early identification of patients at risk. Spine 2014;39:2024–2033
10. Lao L, Weng X, Qiu G, Shen J. The role of preoperative pulmonary function tests in the surgical treatment of extremely severe scoliosis. J Orthop Surg Res 2013;8:32
11. Zhang JG, Wang W, Qiu GX, Wang YP, Weng XS, Xu HG. The role of preoperative pulmonary function tests in the surgical treatment of scoliosis. Spine 2005;30(2):218–221
12. Kelly MP, Zebala LP, Kim HJ, et al; International Spine Study Group. Effectiveness of preoperative autologous

blood donation for protection against allogeneic blood exposure in adult spinal deformity surgeries: a propensity-matched cohort analysis. J Neurosurg Spine 2016;24:124–130

13. Yang B, Li H, Wang D, He X, Zhang C, Yang P. Systematic review and meta-analysis of perioperative intravenous tranexamic acid use in spinal surgery. PLoS One 2013;8:e55436

14. Lenke LG, Bridwell KH, O'Brien MF, Baldus C, Blanke K. Recognition and treatment of the proximal thoracic curve in adolescent idiopathic scoliosis treated with Cotrel-Dubousset instrumentation. Spine 1994; 19:1589–1597

15. Ilharreborde B, Even J, Lefevre Y, et al. How to determine the upper level of instrumentation in Lenke types 1 and 2 adolescent idiopathic scoliosis: a prospective study of 132 patients. J Pediatr Orthop 2008;28:733–739

16. Sharma S, Andersen T, Wu C, et al. How well do radiological assessments of truncal and shoulder balance correlate with cosmetic assessment indices in Lenke 1C adolescent idiopathic scoliosis? Clin Spine Surg 2016;29:341–351

17. Horton WC, Brown CW, Bridwell KH, Glassman SD, Suk SI, Cha CW. Is there an optimal patient stance for obtaining a lateral 36" radiograph? A critical comparison of three techniques. Spine 2005;30:427–433

18. Clements DH, Marks M, Newton PO, Betz RR, Lenke L, Shufflebarger H; Harms Study Group. Did the Lenke classification change scoliosis treatment? Spine 2011;36:1142–1145

19. Cheung KM, Luk KD. Prediction of correction of scoliosis with use of the fulcrum bending radiograph. J Bone Joint Surg Am 1997;79:1144–1150

20. Cheung KM, Natarajan D, Samartzis D, Wong YW, Cheung WY, Luk KD. Predictability of the fulcrum bending radiograph in scoliosis correction with alternate-level pedicle screw fixation. J Bone Joint Surg Am 2010;92:169–176

21. Cheung WY, Lenke LG, Luk KD. Prediction of scoliosis correction with thoracic segmental pedicle screw constructs using fulcrum bending radiographs. Spine 2010;35:557–561

22. Luk KD, Don AS, Chong CS, Wong YW, Cheung KM. Selection of fusion levels in adolescent idiopathic scoliosis using fulcrum bending prediction: a prospective study. Spine 2008;33:2192–2198

23. Hamzaoglu A, Ozturk C, Aydogan M, Tezer M, Aksu N, Bruno MB. Posterior only pedicle screw instrumentation with intraoperative halo-femoral traction in the surgical treatment of severe scoliosis (>100 degrees). Spine 2008;33:979–983

24. Zhang HQ, Gao QL, Ge L, et al. Strong halo-femoral traction with wide posterior spinal release and three dimensional spinal correction for the treatment of severe adolescent idiopathic scoliosis. Chin Med J (Engl) 2012;125:1297–1302

25. Bitan FD, Veliskakis KP, Campbell BC. Differences in the Risser grading systems in the United States and France. Clin Orthop Relat Res 2005;436:190–195

26. Greulich WW, Pyle SI. Radiographic Atlas of Skeletal Development of the Hand and Wrist, 2nd ed. Palo Alto, CA: Stanford University Press; 1959

27. Sanders JO, Browne RH, McConnell SJ, Margraf SA, Cooney TE, Finegold DN. Maturity assessment and curve progression in girls with idiopathic scoliosis. J Bone Joint Surg Am 2007;89:64–73

28. Luk KD, Saw LB, Grozman S, Cheung KM, Samartzis D. Assessment of skeletal maturity in scoliosis patients to determine clinical management: a new classification scheme using distal radius and ulna radiographs. Spine J 2014;14:315–325

29. Winter RB, Lonstein JE, Heithoff KB, Kirkham JA. Magnetic resonance imaging evaluation of the adolescent patient with idiopathic scoliosis before spinal instrumentation and fusion: A prospective, double-blinded study of 140 patients. Spine 1976;97:855–858

4

Late Sequelae of Untreated Pediatric Deformity

Sergio Mendoza-Lattes and Faisal Konbaz

Introduction

There is significant variability in the clinical presentation of adults with untreated pediatric deformity. In longitudinal studies on the natural history of late-onset idiopathic scoliosis, these patients have relatively limited disability compared with unaffected controls.[1–3] However, late sequelae of untreated pediatric deformity may also include symptomatic adult deformity, which can compromise health-related quality of life, particularly in the domains of pain and function, social roles, and mental health.[4,5] This significant and measurable compromise in health-related quality of life can be perceived as comparable or even worse than that of other chronic conditions such as diabetes, chronic lung disease, and congestive heart failure.[4,5] Patients dealing with the variability and uncertainty of the late sequelae of untreated scoliosis often make frequent visits to an adult spine surgery practice, and they express the following concerns: "Am I going to be disabled?" "If I get pregnant, is this going to worsen the scoliosis curve?" "Are my lungs being crushed by the curve?" "Am I going to end up deformed and hunched?" This chapter addresses these questions. Accurate information regarding the natural history of untreated pediatric deformity will empower patients and physicians to make informed choices regarding treatment options.

Curve Progression in Adolescent Idiopathic Scoliosis

The most rapid curve progression in adolescent idiopathic scoliosis (AIS) occurs during the adolescent growth spurt. After skeletal maturity, curve progression is typically noticed over a period of decades rather than months or years. In a longitudinal 40.5-year follow-up study of 102 patients with untreated idiopathic scoliosis, Weinstein and Ponseti[1] found evidence of curve progression after skeletal maturity in 68% of the curves (**Fig. 4.1**). Patients who reach skeletal maturity with curves measuring < 30 degrees can be reassured that their curve is unlikely to progress in adult life. On the other hand, patients with curves measuring ≥ 50 degrees, particularly patients with thoracic curves between 50 and 75 degrees, should be followed periodically because they are more likely to continue to progress.[1,6] With advanced spinal degeneration, curves that have reached 80 to 90 degrees tend to stabilize and progress less rapidly. This is likely related to ankylosis of the apex of the curve, increased rigidity due to the effects of spinal degeneration, and "stability" provided by the rib cage contact with the ilium[6] (**Fig. 4.1**).

Thoracic curves undergo the fastest rate of curve progression, especially curves measuring

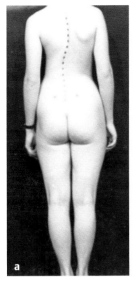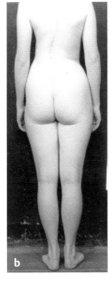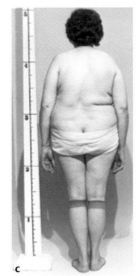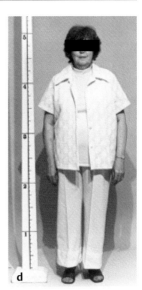

Fig. 4.1 Adolescent idiopathic scoliosis natural history and curve progression. **(a)** Age 14, 40 degrees. **(b)** Age 16, 48 degrees. **(c,d)** Age 69, 90 degrees. (Courtesy of Stuart Weinstein, MD, University of Iowa Department of Orthopaedic Surgery and Rehabilitation.)

between 50 and 75 degrees. The average rate of progression is ~ 1 degree per year of life. For this reason, patients who reach skeletal maturity with curves > 50 degrees should be considered for surgical intervention[1,2,6] (**Fig. 4.2**). Thoracolumbar and lumbar curves > 30 degrees tend to progress, but at a slower rate than thoracic curves, with an average progression rate of 0.5 degree per year of life. These curves have a higher potential to develop translational or rotatory listhesis, a factor commonly associated with pain symptoms.[1,2,6] In particular, lumbar curves commonly develop lateral listhesis at L3-L4 and L4-L5, a frequent cause of radiculopathy in these patients.[7] Although thoracic curves may progress more, lumbar curves are more likely to become symptomatic and lead to the need for surgical care. Finally, double major curves tend to be better balanced with age, and they demonstrate preserved coronal compensation.

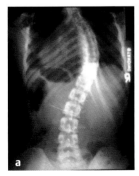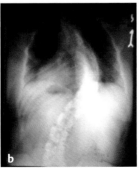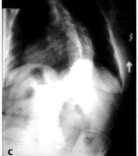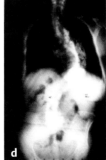

Fig. 4.2 Adolescent idiopathic scoliosis natural history and curve progression. **(a)** Age 21, 53 degrees. **(b)** Age 43, 63 degrees. **(c)** Age 53, 86 degrees. **(d)** Age 66, 94 degrees. (Courtesy of Stuart Weinstein, MD, University of Iowa Department of Orthopaedic Surgery and Rehabilitation.) Weinstein SL, Ponseti IV. Curve progression in idiopathic scoliosis. J Bone Joint Surg Am 1983;65:447–455.)

Cardiopulmonary Sequelae

Late cardiopulmonary compromise is the most concerning potential consequence of untreated scoliosis. Scoliosis is a complex three-dimensional deformity of the spine that can also affect the geometry and range of motion of the chest wall.[8] The respiratory muscles are placed at a biomechanical disadvantage, resulting in decreased chest wall compliance and restrictive lung problems.[9] Autopsy studies have shown evidence of restrictive lung disease in patients with severe spinal deformities,[2] including small airway disease, atelectasis, and sometimes lung atrophy.[10] The abnormal thoracic anatomy may also lead to distortion of the bronchial tree and even to direct compression of bronchi, resulting in extensive areas of hypoventilation.[9]

Pulmonary function impairment secondary to thoracic or thoracolumbar scoliosis curves is proportional to the magnitude and rigidity of the curve, and to the severity of thoracic hypokyphosis.[6,8,10–12] In the Iowa 50-year follow-up natural history cohort,[3] 22% of patients reported shortness of breath with activities of daily living. This was significantly more prevalent with curves > 80 degrees. These results are also reflected in a recent cross-sectional study of 492 patients with scoliosis (94% AIS), of which 10% had evidence of severe restrictive lung disease (forced vital capacity < 50%).[13] This group had significantly larger thoracolumbar curves (80 degrees in the severe impairment group versus 57 degrees in rest of the patients), and these curves were also significantly stiffer (flexibility of 29% in the severe impairment group versus 46% in the rest of the patients). A 20-year follow-up study of patients with untreated scoliosis also supports these conclusions, and further concludes that the percentage of decline in vital capacity (VC) is the strongest predictor of respiratory failure.[14]

Abnormalities in pulmonary function tests reflecting restrictive lung disease can be observed in adult patients with even just moderate curves (40–60 degrees).[15] Although these patients may present with normal blood gas levels at rest, they also have marked abnormalities of gas exchange during exercise, resulting in hypoxemia and hypercapnia.[16,17]

The age of onset of the scoliosis plays an important role in developing cardiopulmonary failure. Excluding neuromuscular disorders, patient who develop cardiorespiratory failure are predominantly those whose curves were first noted prior to the age of 5 years.[18] Curve severity has an effect on lung development and function, particularly prior to the age of 8 years, with a negative effect on the growth and number of alveoli.[16] Patients with AIS are very unlikely to develop respiratory failure regardless of severity.

Pulmonary rehabilitation and respiratory and peripheral muscle training are necessary to increase the endurance and walking distance in these patients.[19] In extreme cases, noninvasive mechanical ventilation (NIMV) results in improved survival.[17]

Childbearing

Despite patient concerns, childbearing does not seem to affect curve progression, regardless of curve location.[20,21] Scoliosis curve progression is similar among women with one or more pregnancies.

Low back pain during pregnancy is common, particularly during the third trimester. This symptom presents at rates similar to those for women without scoliosis.[22] In those with scoliosis, the curve type does not influence the occurrence of back pain. No increased complications of birth and delivery are found in patients with scoliosis, and the rate of cesarean sections is comparable to that in women without scoliosis.[21]

Spondylosis, Back Pain, and Radiculopathy

Back pain is relatively uncommon in adolescents with AIS, but the discussion on whether untreated scoliosis is associated with back pain in adult life is often raised by the patients and their families. The Iowa 50-year follow-up natural history study of 109 patients with untreated scoliosis compared with an age- and sex-matched control cohort provides the most accurate assessment of back pain in patients with untreated scoliosis.[3] Although no difference was found in the intensity or duration of pain symptoms, patients with untreated scoliosis were more likely to present episodes of acute or chronic back pain compared with the control group (61% vs 35%, respectively).[3] This observation is also supported by other longitudinal studies.[9,12,15,22,23] Pain can be generated from the many common disease processes involved in spinal degeneration and pain. These include facet arthropathy, disk degeneration, muscle fatigue, coronal or sagittal imbalance, and foraminal or central stenosis. Curve location has a stronger influence on the development of back pain than the curve magnitude. Thoracolumbar/lumbar curves are more likely associated with back pain than are thoracic curve patterns.[10,15,23]

When evaluating adult patients with symptomatic scoliosis, it is often difficult to determine if these curves are generated de novo (adult degenerative scoliosis) or whether they are AIS curves that have progressed after skeletal maturity. As these curves progress, they also become more rigid, and the ability of the patient to control the alignment of the trunk can be lost. This can result in an unbalanced spine. The factor that seems to be most clearly associated with painful spinal deformity is the presence of sagittal plane imbalance.[24] Coronal imbalance is usually well tolerated when < 4 cm. Patients who do not appear unbalanced and who resort to compensatory mechanisms, such as pelvic retroversion, also have decreased function and quality of life.[25] Finally, translational or rotatory listhesis in the lumbar spine is also more frequently found in symptomatic patients[1,2,6] (**Fig. 4.3**).

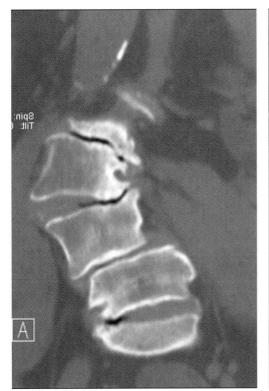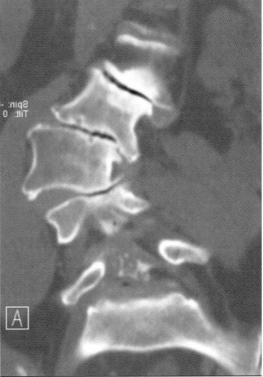

Fig. 4.3 Example of translational or rotatory listhesis commonly found in adult degenerative scoliosis and associated with more frequent pain symptoms. Note the chronic adaptive changes as well as the vacuum phenomena suggesting instability.

Approximately 10% of adults with scoliosis present with radiculopathy symptoms.[10,15] Patients who present with sciatic pain distribution are most likely to have symptomatic foraminal stenosis at the side of the concavity of the caudal fractional curve,[26,27] whereas this is most likely to occur at the concavity of the lumbar structural curve in patients with femoral nerve pain distribution.

Lumbar curves are also associated with higher radiological findings of osteoarthritis at long-term follow-up. The Iowa 50-year longitudinal studies confirm that up to 88% of scoliosis patients with lumbar curves also have radiological evidence of osteoarthritis. At the same time, no significant association between these radiological features and the development of back pain has been found.[2,3]

Quality of Life

Despite having higher prevalence of back pain, most patients with untreated idiopathic scoliosis are able to work and perform activities of daily living at a similar level to that of the general population. By closely following patients with untreated scoliosis for over 50 years, the Iowa studies showed that these patients can function at the level of matched nonscoliosis adults, become employed, get married, and have children. These conclusions are also supported by other 20+-year follow-up studies of patients with AIS treated by bracing.[20,28] Unfortunately, untreated patients can continue to develop significant deformity and are generally dissatisfied with their physical appearance; 32% of these patients feel that their life is limited because of the scoliosis.[3,28]

Mortality

Excluding patients with neuromuscular or genetic conditions, mortality is significantly increased in patients with severe scoliosis curves (> 70 degrees), but almost exclusively in those with early-onset scoliosis.[23] Curve severity has an effect on lung development and function, particularly prior to age 8, with a negative effect on the growth and number of alveoli.[16] Thus, increased mortality is almost exclusively secondary to respiratory failure.[23] Adolescent-onset curves do not have the same impact on mortality, even when severe. A 60-year follow-up on a group of 130 patients supports these conclusions.[23]

▦ Chapter Summary

- Pulmonary function impairment secondary to thoracic or thoracolumbar scoliosis curves is proportional to the magnitude and rigidity of the curve, and to the severity of thoracic hypokyphosis.
- The age of onset of the scoliosis plays an important role in developing cardiopulmonary failure, being most common in those whose curves were first noted prior to the age of 5 years.
- Patients with untreated scoliosis are more likely to present episodes of acute or chronic back pain compared with nonscoliosis individuals, but have a comparable level of function.
- Childbearing does not affect curve progression.
- Mortality is significantly increased in patients with severe scoliosis curves (> 70 degrees), but almost exclusively in those with early-onset scoliosis.

Pearls

- ◆ Understand the natural history of curve progression, particularly in patients with curves > 50 degrees.
- ◆ Restrictive lung disease is evident in pulmonary function tests with curves > 40 degrees, and may become symptomatic with curves > 80 degrees.
- ◆ Childbearing does not affect curve progression.

> **Pitfall**
>
> ◆ Although patients with untreated scoliosis are more likely to present episodes of acute or chronic back pain compared with nonscoliosis individuals, do not attribute all episodes of back pain to the scoliotic curvature.

References

Five Must-Read References

1. Weinstein SL, Ponseti IV. Curve progression in idiopathic scoliosis. J Bone Joint Surg Am 1983;65:447–455

2. Weinstein SL, Zavala DC, Ponseti IV. Idiopathic scoliosis: long-term follow-up and prognosis in untreated patients. J Bone Joint Surg Am 1981;63:702–712

3. Weinstein SL, Dolan LA, Spratt KF, Peterson KK, Spoonamore MJ, Ponseti IV. Health and function of patients with untreated idiopathic scoliosis: a 50-year natural history study. JAMA 2003;289:559–567

4. Pellisé F, Vila-Casademunt A, Ferrer M, et al; European Spine Study Group, ESSG. Impact on health related quality of life of adult spinal deformity (ASD) compared with other chronic conditions. Eur Spine J 2015;24:3–11

5. Bess S, Line B, Fu KM, et al; International Spine Study Group. The Health impact of symptomatic adult spinal deformity: comparison of deformity types to United States population norms and chronic diseases. Spine 2016;41:224–233

6. Agabegi SS, Kazemi N, Sturm PF, Mehlman CT. Natural history of adolescent idiopathic scoliosis in skeletally mature patients: A critical review. J Am Acad Orthop Surg 2015;23:714–723

7. Marty-Poumarat C, Scattin L, Marpeau M, Garreau de Loubresse C, Aegerter P. History of progressive adult scoliosis. Natural Spine 2007;32:1227–1234

8. Qiabi M, Chagnon K, Beaupré A, Hercun J, Rakovich G. Scoliosis and bronchial obstruction. Can Respir J 2015;22:206–208

9. Leong JC, Lu WW, Luk KD, Karlberg EM. Kinematics of the chest cage and spine during breathing in healthy individuals and in patients with adolescent idiopathic scoliosis. Spine 1999;24:1310–1315

10. Barrios C, Pérez-Encinas C, Maruenda JI, Laguía M. Significant ventilatory functional restriction in adolescents with mild or moderate scoliosis during maximal exercise tolerance test. Spine 2005;30:1610–1615

11. Johari J, Sharifudin MA, Ab Rahman A, et al. Relationship between pulmonary function and degree of spinal deformity, location of apical vertebrae and age among adolescent idiopathic scoliosis patients. Singapore Med J 2016;57:33–38

12. Koumbourlis AC. Scoliosis and the respiratory system. Paediatr Respir Rev 2006;7:152–160

13. Dreimann M, Hoffmann M, Kossow K, Hitzl W, Meier O, Koller H. Scoliosis and chest cage deformity measures predicting impairments in pulmonary function: a cross-sectional study of 492 patients with scoliosis to improve the early identification of patients at risk. Spine 2014;39:2024–2033

14. Pehrsson K, Bake B, Larsson S, Nachemson A. Lung function in adult idiopathic scoliosis: a 20 year follow up. Thorax 1991;46:474–478

15. Jackson RP, Simmons EH, Stripinis D. Coronal and sagittal plane spinal deformities correlating with back pain and pulmonary function in adult idiopathic scoliosis. Spine 1989;14:1391–1397

16. Reid L. Lung growth. Proceedings of a Third Symposium held at The Institute of Diseases of the Chest, Brampton Hospital, London, 1970

17. Gustafson T, Franklin KA, Midgren B, Pehrsson K, Ranstam J, Ström K. Survival of patients with kyphoscoliosis receiving mechanical ventilation or oxygen at home. Chest 2006;130:1828–1833

18. Branthwaite MA. Cardiorespiratory consequences of unfused idiopathic scoliosis. Br J Dis Chest 1986;80:360–369

19. Fuschillo S, De Felice A, Martucci M, et al. Pulmonary rehabilitation improves exercise capacity in subjects with kyphoscoliosis and severe respiratory impairment. Respir Care 2015;60:96–101

20. Danielsson AJ, Wiklund I, Pehrsson K, Nachemson AL. Health-related quality of life in patients with adolescent idiopathic scoliosis: a matched follow-up at least 20 years after treatment with brace or surgery. Eur Spine J 2001;10:278–288

21. Danielsson AJ, Nachemson AL. Childbearing, curve progression, and sexual function in women 22 years after treatment for adolescent idiopathic scoliosis: a case-control study. Spine 2001;26:1449–1456

22. Cordover AM, Betz RR, Clements DH, Bosacco SJ. Natural history of adolescent thoracolumbar and lumbar

idiopathic scoliosis into adulthood. J Spinal Disord 1997;10:193–196

23. Pehrsson K, Larsson S, Oden A, Nachemson A. Long-term follow-up of patients with untreated scoliosis. A study of mortality, causes of death, and symptoms. Spine 1992;17:1091–1096

24. Glassman SD, Berven S, Bridwell K, Horton W, Dimar JR. Correlation of radiographic parameters and clinical symptoms in adult scoliosis. Spine 2005;30: 682–688

25. Lafage V, Schwab F, Patel A, Hawkinson N, Farcy JP. Pelvic tilt and truncal inclination: two key radiographic parameters in the setting of adults with spinal deformity. Spine 2009;34:E599–E606

26. Haefeli M, Elfering A, Kilian R, Min K, Boos N. Nonoperative treatment for adolescent idiopathic scoliosis:

a 10- to 60-year follow-up with special reference to health-related quality of life. Spine 2006;31:355–366, discussion 367

27. Pugely AJ, Ries Z, Gnanapragasam G, Gao Y, Nash R, Mendoza-Lattes S. Curve characteristics and foraminal dimensions in patients with adult scoliosis and radiculopathy. Clin Spine Surge 2016; [Epub ahead of print]

28. Weinstein SL, Dolan LA. The evidence base for the prognosis and treatment of adolescent idiopathic scoliosis: The 2015 Orthopaedic Research and Education Foundation Clinical Research Award. J Bone Joint Surg Am 2015;97:1899–1903

5

Surgical Techniques for the Management of Early-Onset Scoliosis

Joshua S. Murphy, Burt Yaszay, and Behrooz A. Akbarnia

Introduction

Management of early-onset scoliosis (EOS) presents a difficult challenge in pediatric spine surgery. Since Harrington first introduced instrumentation without fusion in 27 post-polio and idiopathic patients, growing rod techniques have continued to evolve from one rod and two hooks with subperiosteal dissection to magnetically controlled growing rods that can be lengthened in the clinic and may only require one operative procedure requiring anesthesia.[1,2]

As we continue to learn more about the natural history of EOS, our surgical techniques and goals have continued to evolve. In this paradigm shift, a short, straight spine is no longer acceptable. However, some spine deformity is acceptable if spine and chest growth can be maintained, allowing more normal cardiopulmonary development and function. Furthermore, multiple techniques have been described to treat EOS, as one general technique cannot be used for all patients. The surgeon must choose the appropriate technique for each patient, to provide the best possible outcome not only in curve correction, but also in cardiopulmonary development and future growth, and with the least risk of complications.

This chapter describes various growth-friendly surgical techniques in the management of EOS, primarily the distraction techniques using traditional growing rods, magnetically controlled growing rods, and vertical expandable prosthetic titanium ribs, as well as growth guidance techniques such as the Shilla and Luque trolley. Growth modulation, including anterior vertebral body stapling and anterior vertebral body tethering, is discussed in a subsequent chapter, as it is not commonly used in EOS.

Single and Dual Traditional Growing Rods

The growing rod technique is most appropriate in patients with idiopathic, neuromuscular, or syndromic scoliosis in the absence of congenital anomalies. Fairly comparable results have been reported for the use of the dual-rod technique for congenital deformities in patients who still have some growth potential.[3] The growing rod may not be an effective procedure when there is no further growth potential or in patients whose primary problem is chest wall abnormalities or thoracic insufficiency syndrome. The use of both single and dual growing rod constructs can be considered a useful adjunct in the treatment of severe progressive spinal deformities in EOS.

Surgical Technique for Single Growing Rods (Fig. 5.1)

Although the dual growing rod has been shown to be a more stable construct in general, the single-rod technique continues to be utilized for some patients with EOS.[4–6] In cases where the patient is small and the skin is tenuous, the rod may be prominent over the convex side of the curve, the single-rod technique provides a lower profile construct. As with all growing rod techniques, meticulous preoperative planning and attention to detail is paramount to obtaining a good outcome.

This is our preferred technique: The patient is brought to the operating room, connected to neuromonitoring, and placed under general anesthesia. Prophylactic antibiotics are administered prior to the start of the procedure, and the back is prepped and draped in sterile fashion. Typically, a midline skin incision is made over the portion of the spine to be instrumented. With use of meticulous hemostasis, the fascia is exposed at the levels of the proximal and distal foundations. We then expose one spinous process proximal and one distal, and mark them with a clamp. Intraoperative imaging is utilized to identify the preplanned foundation sites. Once identified, the two to three adjacent vertebrae are exposed subperiosteally to be used as the foundation on the concave aspect of the curve. The fascia between the proximal and distal foundations is preserved, and a rod is passed on the concave side subfascially, typically from distal to proximal. Once this is complete, work begins on the distal foundation site utilizing a pedicle screw construct, as we believe this provides a more solid distal foundation. The proximal foundation consists of a claw construct, with an over-the-top laminar hook proximally and a sublaminar hook in the next distal vertebrae. This enables compression between the hooks once the rod has been inserted. On occasion, this may be extended one level distal. At times, if a hook construct is unable to be utilized one can also consider

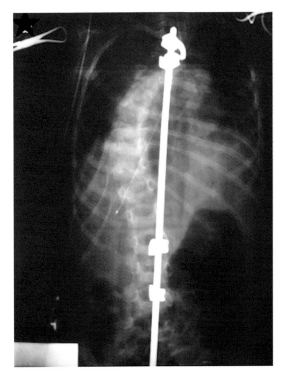 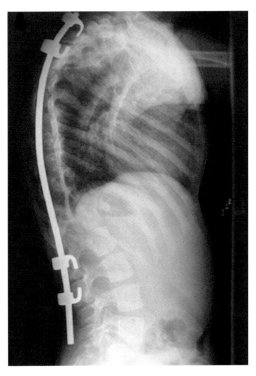

a

Fig. 5.1 Postoperative anteroposterior **(a)** and lateral **(b)** radiographs of a patient who underwent a Shilla procedure for early-onset scoliosis (EOS). (Courtesy of Scott J. Luhmann, MD.)

an all-pedicle-screw construct for the proximal foundation. The size of the rod is determined by the size of the patient. In most small children, a 4.5- to 5.5-mm titanium rod is used, whereas in older children, a larger diameter rod may be utilized. When measuring the rod, typically allow for an additional 5 to 6 cm to compensate for initial distraction, and allow enough extra length to enable it to be expanded at subsequent surgeries. The rod is contoured to the desired sagittal plane. Once inserted, it is grasped with rod holders and rotated to correct and align the sagittal plane. The upper foundation is typically tightened first and the rod is distracted distally. There should be 4 to 5 cm of rod extended below the distal hook or screw to be used for subsequent lengthenings. The wound is irrigated with normal saline solution and closed in layers.

Although this is our preferred technique, different variations of techniques have been developed over time, including those using anchors bilaterally of the proximal and distal foundations connected with a cross-link, creating a more stable foundation and using only one rod along the concavity of the curve. This technique may provide better control of spinal rotation than would be provided by a one-sided foundation. This is an interesting technique that may be considered when utilizing a single-rod technique.

Surgical Technique for Dual Growing Rods (Fig. 5.2)

The setup is similar to that described above for a single growing rod. The index procedure can typically be performed through one or two midline incisions.[7,8] Clamps are placed on the spinous processes once they are exposed and once the levels have been verified under image intensification. Meticulous technique is used to avoid a broad exposure and risk spontaneous fusion. Exposures at the foundations are the only locations used to perform a subperiosteal dissection.

The upper foundation is generally placed between the levels of T2 to T4. In a typical dual-rod construct, we utilize at least four anchors (hooks and screws) for each foundation for maximum stability. Our preference is to use four hooks at the upper foundation. Harrington's[1] preference is a supralaminar hook for the superior location and a sublaminar hook under the lamina, creating a bilateral claw construct. Occasionally, in patients with a small transverse diameter of the spinal column, there is concern about crowding the spinal canal, causing canal stenosis. In these cases, the hooks can be staggered over two to three levels. If this is the case, one must remember that the hooks may block the use of a transverse connector at the proximal foundation level. In that event, the connector can be placed just caudad to the lower hooks. Although our preference is hooks, occasionally hooks are difficult to place secondary to the patient's anatomy, and in those cases we utilize a pedicle screw construct. Mahar et al[8] demonstrated an increased stability of pedicle screws over hooks alone. We therefore always use transverse connectors when using proximal hooks. In the event that proximal pedicle screws are warranted, care must be taken with placement, especially in hyperkyphotic patients, as cutout into the spinal canal can be catastrophic.

The caudal foundation is typically instrumented with four pedicle screws. The lowest instrumented vertebra (LIV) of the foundation tends to be the most proximal horizontal lumbar vertebra. However, the goal is to avoid instrumenting to the pelvis in ambulatory patients. It is important to create a strong, stable foundation. Therefore, a combination of local bone autograft and cancellous chips allograft with demineralized bone matrix is used to augment the bony fusion across the foundation sites. Once the foundations have been adequately prepared, a low-profile implant system is chosen. These are often two 4.5-mm titanium or stainless steel rods. The rods are measured and cut into four segments. The two proximal rods (one for the left and one for the right) are contoured with the appropriate kyphosis. The two distal rods are contoured with the appropriate lumbar lordosis. One proximal and one distal rod are connected with a straight box connector that usually spans the thoracolumbar junction. Appropriate contouring may help to correct the sagittal

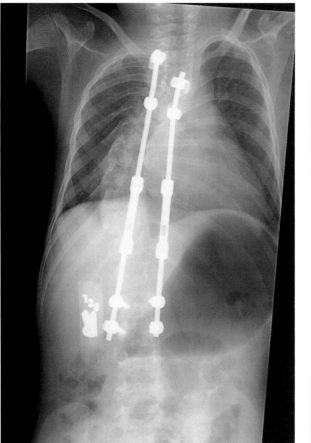

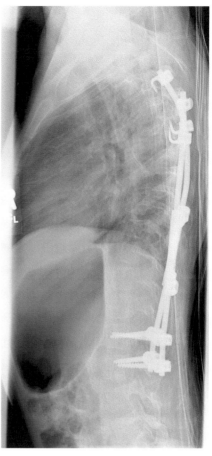

a

Fig. 5.2 Anteroposterior (**a**) and lateral (**b**) radiographs of a patient with EOS who underwent placement of a growth-friendly dual growing rod construct. (Courtesy of Michael L. Schmitz, MD.)

plane deformity and restore it to a more normal profile in a flexible curve. However, one must be careful to avoid extreme sagittal correction, as this may lead to anchor failure especially in stiffer curves. At this point, the rods are passed subfascially from the caudal to cephalad direction while palpating the tip of the rod so as to avoid penetration into the pleural cavity. The rod is secured to the anchors. As previously mentioned, if an all-hook construct is utilized at the cephalad foundation, it is strongly recommended to use a cross connector. The cross connector is not necessary if using a four-pedicle-screw construct.

When a tandem connector is used for periodic lengthening, the majority of lengthenings are completed by loosening the screw of the upper rod. Therefore, only a short segment of the lower rod is secured to the tandem connector. The segment of the rods entering the connector should not be contoured, as the connector is straight and this will create a stress riser at the transition and also may interfere with smooth lengthening. The tandem connectors are placed in the least prominent position of the thoracolumbar region to achieve a low-profile construct. If set screws are used with tandem connectors, they can be positioned either medially or laterally. The benefit of placing the screws medially is that they can be accessed more easily in a less invasive fashion during future lengthening procedures. However, lateral placement may have a lower profile in a very small child. At this point, the initial correction and lengthening can be performed. Extreme care must be taken so as not to over-distract, leading to immediate implant or neurologic complication. During the initial surgery, care is taken so as not to maximally distract across the deformity. We tend to wait until the first distraction when the foundation fusions are more mature, and then prefer not distracting more than 2 cm because of concern about inadvertently causing a neurologic injury.

Traditional growing rod lengthening procedures are typically performed every 6 to 9 months. In healthy children, this can be performed on an outpatient basis or during a short hospital stay. However, children with significant medical comorbidities may require an inpatient or even an intensive care unit stay. We choose to use intraoperative neuromonitoring for all growing rod procedures including lengthenings. Sankar et al[9] conducted a multicenter retrospective review of 782 growing rod surgeries (252 growing rod implantations, 168 implant exchanges, and 362 lengthenings) in 252 patients. They identified neuromonitoring changes in two patients during primary implantation, one during implant exchange and one during lengthening. Furthermore, Akbarnia et al[10] reported a case of delayed neurologic deficit after a rod exchange procedure despite normal somatosensory evoked potentials (SSEPs), Hoffman reflexes, and electromyograms (EMGs) intraoperatively. The patient made a full recovery after shortening of the rod.

For dual-rod lengthening, a small midline incision is made centered between the tandem connectors at the site of the rod gap. The skin incision is made to the depth of the tandem connector prior to working laterally, so as to maintain the integrity of the overlying skin and soft tissue coverage. Both connectors are exposed, and the upper set screws are loosened. The rod on the side of the spine needing the most length, usually the concavity, is distracted first. A rod holder is placed on the rod, and the lengthening over the rod is performed by distracting between the rod holder and the connector. The same technique is used for lengthening of the contralateral side. Typically, the distraction is performed to match the first side. As with the index procedure, care must be taken not to over-distract the rods during lengthenings.

Vertical Expandable Prosthetic Titanium Rib Expansion Thoracoplasty (Fig. 5.3)

Thoracic insufficiency syndrome (TIS) is considered the inability of the thorax to support normal respiration and lung growth.[11,12] The natural history of the syndrome has a high mortality in cases of untreated early-onset spine and chest wall deformity. TIS is the primary indication for vertical expandable prosthetic titanium rib (VEPTR) expansion thoracoplasty. The Food and Drug Administration (FDA) has approved VEPTR expansion thoracoplasty for the treatment of TIS in the skeletally immature patient. Contraindications to the use of VEPTR are skeletal maturity, poor rib bone stock, and absence of proximal ribs. The general surgical strategy depends on the type of

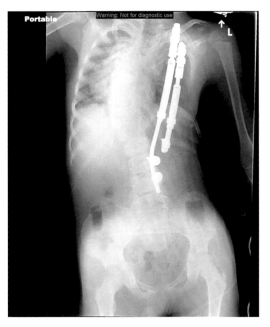

Fig. 5.3 Anteroposterior radiograph of a patient who underwent vertical expandable prosthetic titanium rib (VEPTR) expansion thoracoplasty secondary to thoracic insufficiency syndrome. (Courtesy of Michael L. Schmitz, MD.)

volume depletion deformity. Open-wedge thoracostomy, also known as expansion thoracoplasty, is utilized for unilateral constriction of the thorax. This is the primary focus of this surgical technique.

The general surgical approach and technique are performed with the patient in the prone position. Spinal cord monitoring and prophylactic antibiotics are utilized and maintained for 24 hours postoperatively, or until all drains have been removed. To start, a modified curvilinear thoracotomy incision is made between the ninth and tenth ribs from just lateral to the paraspinous muscles, extending anterior to the costocartilage segments. Be sure to identify the common insertion of the middle and posterior scalene muscles to protect the neurovascular bundle just anterior to them. Once there is complete exposure of the rib cage, the paraspinous muscles are reflected medially to the tips of the transverse processes with great care taken so as not to expose the spine and prevent inadvertent fusion. The lengthened hemithorax is stabilized by a hybrid VEPTR device from the proximal to distal direction to avoid penetrating the chest and causing cardiopulmonary injury. Of note, in patients under the age of 18 months, a single rib-to-rib VEPTR is used secondary to inadequate spinal canal width, precluding the use a spinal hook. When the patient reaches 2 to 3 years of age, the VEPTR can be converted to a hybrid construct from the proximal ribs to the lumbar spine. Depending on the size of the thoracic cavity, a second VEPTR can be placed, or a VEPTR gantry construct using transverse bars and right-angle rib cradles can be placed to increase the overall surface area and load share the device. The second device can be placed laterally in the posterior axillary line. If areas of chest wall instability are noted more anteriorly, additional rib-to-rib VEPTR devices can be added as needed, taking care to position them well below the neurovascular bundle.

At this point, the equilibrium of the thorax should be obtained as much as possible in all planes to maximize the space available for the lungs. Prior to starting the closure, the scapula should be brought down to its approximate anatomic location, the arm is elevated over the head, and SSEPs are checked for signs of acute thoracic outlet syndrome. If an anomalous rib is present it can be pushed into the brachial plexus by the expansion thoracoplasty. Findings include decreased signal in the ulnar nerve distribution and diminished pulses. If findings are positive, one can relax the position of the scapula, allowing it to settle in a more proximal position. If this does not work, it may be necessary to resect the anterolateral portions of the first and second ribs lateral to the VEPTR to provide space for the VEPTR in the newly reconstructed thorax.[12]

Once the VEPTR devices are in place, the muscle and skin flaps are stretched to provide adequate soft tissue coverage for the expanded hemithorax. Two subcutaneous drains are placed, and the tissues closed in layers. The drains are typically left in place until the amount draining tapers off to less than 50 cc over a 24-hour period. Bracing is typically not required because of its constrictive effects, and patients are mobilized as soon as possible.

Magnetically Controlled Growing Rods (Fig. 5.4)

There is currently only one FDA-approved magnetically controlled growing rod (MCGR) available in the United States—the MAGEC (NuVasive Inc., San Diego, CA). The device has clearance for the treatment of progressive EOS in immature patients with, or at risk for, TIS. The MAGEC system includes an implantable rod with an adjustable actuator portion with enclosed magnet, manual distractor, magnet locator, and external remote control (ERC) for lengthenings. The implantable rod has two different choices of actuator lengths of 70 mm and 90 mm, which allows for a total of 28 mm and 48 mm of distraction.

Current indications for MCGR are similar to those for traditional growing rods and include the treatment of progressive EOS in immature patients with, or at risk for, TIS. The procedure is contraindicated in patients with infection or pathological conditions that impair secure fixation, in patients with sensitivities to implant materials or with metal allergies, and in patients with a pacemaker or other active electronic

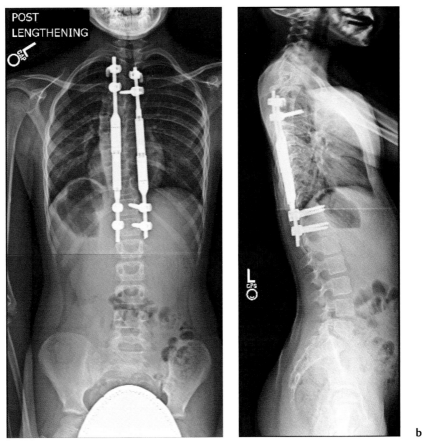

Fig. 5.4 Anteroposterior **(a)** and lateral **(b)** radiographs of a patient who underwent dual magnetically controlled growing rod insertion secondary to EOS. (Courtesy of Michael L. Schmitz, MD.)

device, as well as in patients who are younger than 2 years old or weigh less than 25 lb, or whose family is unable or unwilling to follow postoperative instructions. Magnetic resonance imaging (MRI) is no longer contraindicated in patients with an MCGR, as the FDA has now cleared the device under a special conditions provision.

The technical principles, selection of levels, and preparation of foundation sites of the procedure are similar to those described for the use of traditional growing rods, as previously described in this chapter. Following proper patient positioning, creating a sterile field, and administering preoperative antibiotics, the selected levels are approached through one long or two (one proximal and one distal) midline incisions. Anchors are placed using screws, hooks, bands, or a combination including two or more levels as dictated by the patient's anatomy and surgeon preference. We typically prefer hooks and/or pedicle screws as proximal anchors, and pedicle screws for the distal foundation.

In regard to rod preparation and contouring components for insertion, we prefer to place the actuator between T10 and L2 if possible, where the spine is straight in the sagittal plane. Care should be taken to avoid bending the rod at any point at the actuator or within 20 mm of it because the deformation will preclude the possibility of using the lengthening mechanism. The surgeon should be cautious in patients with excessive kyphosis because of an increased risk of complications due to proximal pullout. If the patient requires extensive contouring or has a small stature, the shorter 70-mm actuator may be used to leave more rod length available for contouring.

Once the rod has been contoured to the needed specifications, it is important to test the actuator and ensure that the actuator lengthens correctly prior to implantation. The manual distractor can be used intraoperatively in sterile fashion to test the actuator. It is recommended to make sure that the provided arrows are pointing toward the cephalad direction, and that four full counterclockwise rotations are performed to ensure the rod is properly functioning. The rod is then returned to a neutral position and prepared for insertion by three clockwise rotations to shorten the rod, but not all the way, to avoid jamming. A standard chest tube can be used to tunnel the rod subfascially between the two foundation sites. The rod can then be passed through the same tunnel. When using dual rods, we prefer to implant the concave rod first for single curves. Both rods are first attached to the proximal foundation, the anchors are preliminarily tightened, and a cross-connector is added between the two rods if necessary. The rods are then connected to the distal foundation loosely. The concave rod is distracted first through the anchor, followed by the convex rod. No cross-link is used distally unless hook anchors are utilized. Of note, when using dual rods, a combination of two single standard rods or a single standard rod and an offset rod can be chosen largely based on surgeon preference and the need for independent rod distraction. A standard and offset combination can be chosen if the surgeon's preference is to distract the rods individually and independently in opposite directions. Regardless of the type of rod, it is suggested to place the actuators at the same cranial/caudal level to obtain the best function. Once placement is verified under image intensification, decortication is performed and the spine is prepared for fusion at the foundations. The soft tissues are closed in layers with a watertight closure.

There is some variation in the methods and frequency of lengthenings. Currently, the ideal method and frequency are not known. Our current preference is for more frequent, such as monthly, lengthenings of ~ 2 mm or lengthenings every other month of 3 mm, as we believe this may decrease the amount of soft tissue trauma and inflammatory response. There are two techniques that can be used when lengthening a dual rod construct: lengthen both rods at the same time or lengthen them individually. It has yet to be determined if one technique is superior to the other.

Growth-Guided Technique: The Shilla Procedure (Fig. 5.5)

The goal of the Shilla procedure is to gain control of the deformity apex, maximize the number of growth centers, and harness the growth potential of the patient by directing the spine into more normal alignment. The concept stemmed from the original Luque trolley technique. The main difference between the Shilla and Luque trolley is that the Shilla causes less periosteal stripping and is thought to lead to less ankylosis and autofusion, allowing more spinal growth and better overall maintenance of correction. In addition, the Shilla derotates and fuses the apical segments, enabling proximal and distal growth, whereas the Luque trolley consists of one pair of rods fixed cephalad and one pair fixed caudad, and the apex is translated without deroration and then captured by the four rods.[13,14]

Preoperative planning consists of analyzing the deformity and flexibility. Determining the location of the apical fusion is of utmost importance. Typically, the three or four vertebrae that show the least correction on bending radiographs will be the levels fused to obtain maximum correction, with the goal of creating neutral alignment in all planes with the fusion. The screws placed at the apex of the curve have a fixed head to provide maximal correction.

The Shilla pedicle screw is a fixed pedicle screw with a locking plug that fixes to the top of the screw and not the rod, allowing the rod to slide in a longitudinal direction through the screw head. These screws are placed cephalad and caudad to the apical fusion to guide the

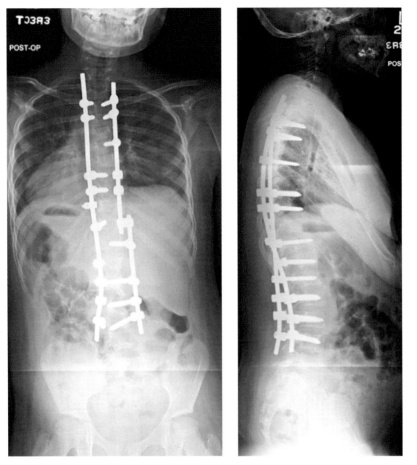

Fig. 5.5 Anteroposterior **(a)** and lateral **(b)** radiographs of a patient who underwent a Shilla procedure for juvenile idiopathic scoliosis.

growth of the spine at the ends of the curve and maintain the coronal and sagittal correction. These screws are placed through a muscular plane without taking down the soft tissues except to cut the fascial planes on each side of the spine. Subperiosteal dissection is limited only to the area of the apical fusion. The choice of local autograft and cancellous chips with demineralized bone matrix are utilized for the fusion.

Once the patient has been placed prone on the table, sterile preparation performed, and prophylactic antibiotics administered, radiographs are obtained with small needle markers placed into the spinous processes to mark the predetermined levels. At the apex, a direct

midline incision is then made with meticulous hemostasis down to the fascia. The fascia is incised 1 cm off the midline on both sides of the spinous processes with subperiosteal dissection. Bilateral fixed-head pedicle screws are placed at the apex. Posterior column osteotomies may be required to assist with full correction, and decortication is performed to fuse these segments.

The Shilla growth guidance screws are placed through the muscular layer without direct visualization, under image guidance. One can use a cannulated polyaxial screw of sufficient diameter to fill the pedicle. The Shilla screws can be placed bilaterally or staggered. However, the surgeon must ensure that they are spread far enough apart to facilitate sliding of the rod. If necessary, in cases when there is concern for screw cutout into the spinal canal, sublaminar wires can be placed cephalad to the proximal screws with minimal dissection, leaving the periosteum and interspinous ligaments intact. Only a small amount of ligamentum flavum needs to be removed to pass the sublaminar wires. A 4.5-mm rod is chosen for smaller children and 5.5-mm rod is chosen for larger children. The rod is contoured to fit a normal sagittal profile and then reduced to the screws. It is one vertebral level long at each end to allow for growth.

The apical segments are derotated and held in place with the rod reduced. The fixed head screws lock the rods at the apical screws using locking set screws, while the Shilla caps proximally and distally capture the rods in the Shilla pedicle screws and provide force on the polyaxial screws and not the rod. If necessary, a cross-link can be placed distally to the proximal foundation to provide additional stability. The soft tissues are closed in layers, and a drain is placed superficial to the fascia. A custom thoracolumbar orthosis is fitted in the hospital to be worn when the patient is out of bed for the first 3 months postoperatively until fusion is complete. At that time, the brace is no longer required. It is important to understand that the 4.5-mm rods generally last 4 to 6 years prior to fracture, and larger 5.5-mm rods may last longer.[15,16]

Novel Techniques

In addition to the more traditional distraction-based and growth guidance techniques, there is growing interest in the use of growth modulation in pediatric spine deformity care. Growth modulation utilizes either staples or screws placed into the anterior vertebral body and uses the spine's inherent growth to correct the deformity by modulating growth of the vertebral body. These techniques are discussed in a subsequent chapter and are not commonly used in a very young child.

Chapter Summary

Growth-friendly surgery is a powerful treatment option for children with EOS, but it is associated with a high risk of complications. The ultimate goal is to improve the quality of life of these children, and the treatment of EOS continues to remain a challenge to the treating surgeon. We believe that one technique cannot be used for all forms of EOS. Therefore, it is important for the surgeon to choose the appropriate technique for each patient, maximizing cardiopulmonary and clinical outcomes while minimizing risks. Our current understanding of the natural history of EOS is limited, and as our knowledge continues to improve, it is likely so will the treatment options. It is important for the surgeon to understand the variety of etiologies that lead to EOS and pay close attention to the patient and the underlying disease.

Pearls

◆ Optimizing patient health, nutrition, and surgical technique along with meticulous handing of soft tissues will decrease the risk of complications.

◆ EOS is a challenging spine and trunk deformity that, depending on the etiology, can affect multiple organ systems, and one technique cannot treat all forms. The surgeon must choose the appropriate technique for each patient.

◆ Early recognition and aggressive treatment of complications, especially infection, may help to mitigate their effects and allow retention of implants.

◆ Ideal indications for TGR: idiopathic, neuromuscular, or syndromic scoliosis and absence of congenital anomalies.

◆ Ideal indications for MCGR: idiopathic, neuromuscular, or syndromic scoliosis and absence of congenital anomalies in patients of at least 2 years of age and weighing 25 lb, with no need for future MRI.

◆ Ideal indications for Shilla: idiopathic, neuromuscular, or syndromic scoliosis with a single curve pattern.

◆ Ideal indications for VEPTR: presence of thoracic insufficiency in a skeletally immature patient with absent ribs, constrictive chest wall syndrome, hypoplastic thorax, or EOS of congenital or neurogenic origin without rib anomaly.

Pitfalls

◆ Be cautious in patients with increased thoracic kyphosis, as they are at an increased risk of proximal anchor pullout. Patients with significant thoracic kyphosis may benefit from preoperative halo traction or release.

◆ Keep subperiosteal dissection only to the areas of the foundation, in an effort to decrease the risk of spontaneous autofusion of the spine, which can limit further spine growth or contribute to a progressive deformity.

◆ Be sure not to over-distract patients during the index procedure or during subsequent lengthenings to decrease the risk of proximal implant failure or neurologic compromise.

References
Five Must-Read References

1. Harrington PR. Treatment of scoliosis. Correction and internal fixation by spine instrumentation. J Bone Joint Surg Am 1962;44-A:591–610

2. Akbarnia BA, Cheung K, Noordeen H, et al. Next generation of growth-sparing techniques: preliminary clinical results of a magnetically controlled growing rod in 14 patients with early-onset scoliosis. Spine 2013;38:665–670

3. Elsebai HB, Yazici M, Thompson GH, et al. Safety and efficacy of growing rod technique for pediatric congenital spinal deformities. J Pediatr Orthop 2011;31:1–5

4. Thompson GH, Akbarnia BA, Kostial P, et al. Comparison of single and dual growing rod techniques followed through definitive surgery: a preliminary study. Spine 2005;30:2039–2044

5. Zhao Y, Qiu GX, Wang YP, et al. Comparison of initial efficacy between single and dual growing rods in treatment of early onset scoliosis. Chin Med J (Engl) 2012;125:2862–2866

6. Akbarnia BA, Marks DS, Boachie-Adjei O, Thompson AG, Asher MA. Dual growing rod technique for the treatment of progressive early-onset scoliosis: a multicenter study. Spine 2005;30(17, Suppl):S46–S57

7. Akbarnia BA, Breakwell LM, Marks DS, et al; Growing Spine Study Group. Dual growing rod technique followed for three to eleven years until final fusion: the effect of frequency of lengthening. Spine 2008;33:984–990

8. Mahar AT, Bagheri R, Oka R, Kostial P, Akbarnia BA. Biomechanical comparison of different anchors (foundations) for the pediatric dual growing rod technique. Spine J 2008;8:933–939

9. Sankar WN, Skaggs DL, Emans JB, et al. Neurologic risk in growing rod spine surgery in early onset scoliosis: is neuromonitoring necessary for all cases? Spine 2009;34:1952–1955

10. Akbarnia BA, et al. Does subcutaneous placement of the rods give better results in growing rod technique? J Child Orthop 2009;3:145–168

11. Campbell RM Jr, Smith MD, Mayes TC, et al. The characteristics of thoracic insufficiency syndrome associated with fused ribs and congenital scoliosis. J Bone Joint Surg Am 2003;85-A:399–408

12. Campbell RM. VEPTR expansion thoracoplasty. In: Akbarnia BA, Yazici M, Thompson GH, eds. The Growing Spine. Management of Spinal Disorders in Young Children. Berlin, Heidelberg: Springer-Verlag; 2016:669–690

13. Luque ER. Treatment of scoliosis without arthrodesis or external support: preliminary report. Clin Orthop Relat Res 1976;119:276

14. McCarthy RE, Luhmann S, Lenke L, McCullough FL. The Shilla growth guidance technique for early-onset spinal deformities at 2-year follow-up: a preliminary report. J Pediatr Orthop 2014;34:1–7

15. Akbarnia BA, Yazici M, Thompson GH, eds. The Growing Spine. Management of Spinal Disorders in Young Children. Berlin, Heidelberg: Springer-Verlag; 2016

16. McCarthy RE, McCullough FL. Shilla growth guidance for early onset scoliosis: results after a minimum of five years follow-up. J Bone Joint Surg Am 2015;97:1578–1584

6

Surgical Techniques for Adolescent Idiopathic Scoliosis and the Selection of Fusion Levels

André Luís Fernandes Andújar, Luis Eduardo Munhoz da Rocha, and Cristiano Magalhães Menezes

▥ Introduction

Following the development of the third-generation implants by Cotrel and Dubousset in the 1980s, which included the use of pedicular screws to the thoracic spine, the King classification[1] became obsolete, making it necessary to develop a new classification system to enable more accurate planning of the surgical treatment of adolescent idiopathic scoliosis (AIS). The Lenke et al classification[2,3] system was then developed to define which curves should be instrumented. However, it does not address the specific fusion levels, such as the upper instrumented vertebra (UIV) and the lower instrumented vertebra (LIV). Suk et al[4] also described another classification system, giving special attention to the definition of the LIV in both thoracic and thoracolumbar or lumbar curves (TL/L). The main objective of the surgical treatment of AIS is the tridimensional correction of the deformity, preserving as many motion segments as possible, and resulting in a balanced trunk in the sagittal and coronal plane with level shoulders. Therefore, choosing the appropriate UIV and LIV is of extreme importance in achieving these goals.

This chapter presents practical rules for defining the fusion levels for each type of curve, based on the literature and on our experience.

▥ Choosing the Levels

Step 1: Which Curves to Include

Once the type of curve has been correctly identified according to the Lenke et al classification system,[2,3] the first rule is to include all the vertebrae of the major curve in the fusion area.[5] It is important to never leave any vertebra of the major curve out of the fusion. The second rule is to include all the secondary structured curves into the fusion. However, there may be some exceptions to this rule, especially in some Lenke 3C and 6C curves where a selective fusion may be done.[5] Even in nonstructured type C TL/L, whether or not to include this curve is controversial.

Step 2: Choosing the Upper Instrumented Vertebra for Thoracic Curves (Lenke 1 to 4)

The goal is to have the shoulders level postoperatively. Initially, the surgeon determines whether or not the proximal thoracic (PT) curve needs to be included in the arthrodesis, based on clinical and radiographic parameters. The PT is included in the following situations:

- The PT is structured (that is, it does not correct to less then 25 degrees in bending films).

- The left shoulder is higher in the clinical evaluation.
- The transition from the PT to the main thoracic (MT) curve is below T5 (these curves are usually structural).[6]
- There is a regional kyphosis between T2 and T5 of more than 25 degrees.

In the presence of any of these criteria, the inclusion of the PT in the fusion is considered; otherwise, the shoulders will rarely correct spontaneously, or there will be a proximal hyperkyphosis that is cosmetically not acceptable. In such cases, the UIV should be T2. To allow a smooth transition from the extremely mobile cervical spine to a rigid and fused thoracic spine, T1 should be avoided as the UIV.

If none of the above criteria is present, there is no need to include the PT in the arthrodesis, and the UIV may be the neutral vertebra (NV) just above the MT, usually the proximal end vertebra (PEV) of the MT or one vertebra above.

Step 3: Choosing the Lower Instrumented Vertebra for Thoracic Curves (Lenke 1 to 4)

Structural Lumbar Curves (Lenke 3 and 4)

When a major MT is accompanied with structured TL/L (Lenke 3 and 4), it is usually neces-sary to include the TL/L in the arthrodesis. In this case, the LIV should be the distal end vertebra (DEV), as will be discussed below. In some Lenke 3C and 4C curves, however, it is possible to perform a selective thoracic fusion, without including the TL/L in the arthrodesis. Making this decision is discussed below about C Modifiers.

Nonstructural Lumbar Curves (Lenke 1 and 2)

If the major MT is accompanied with a non-structured TL/L (Lenke 1 and 2), the choice of LIV is controversial. To facilitate and clarify the selection process, we will discuss the A and B lumbar modifiers and the C modifiers separately.

A and B Modifiers

According to Miyanji et al,[7] the A and B lumbar modifiers are not sufficient to describe different curves for the Lenke type 1 curves. These authors subclassified the 1A curves as 1AL and 1AR (**Fig. 6.1**). In the 1AL curves, the L4 is tilted to the left, whereas in the 1AR curves, the L4 is tilted to the right. The 1AL curves behave similarly to the 1B curves. These concepts can also be used for the Lenke type 2 curves.

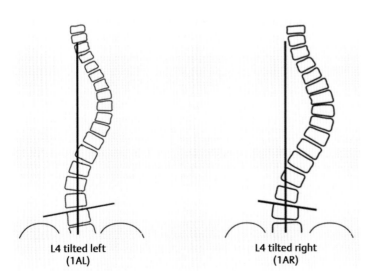

Fig. 6.1 Differentiation between 1AL and 1AR curves based on the direction of L4 tilt. (Reproduced with permission from Miyanji F, Pawelek JB, Van Valin SE, Upasani VV, Newton PO. Is the lumbar modifier useful in surgical decision making?: defining two distinct Lenke 1A curve patterns. Spine 2008;33: 2545–2551.)

L4 tilted left
(1AL)

L4 tilted right
(1AR)

For 1AL and 1B curves, the LIV should be the stable vertebra (SV), but for a 1AR curve, the SV is too distal, making it possible to fuse it shorter.[7] According to Suk et al,[8] the relationship between the DEV and the NV is the best way to define the LIV. When the number of vertebrae between the NV and DEV is 1 or 0, the NV should be chosen as the LIV. When this difference is 2 or more, the LIV may be one vertebra proximal to the NV (NV-1). The LIV should never be two vertebrae above the NV (NV-2) because of the high risk of adding on and decompensation.[8]

C Modifiers

The first step is to decide if it is possible to perform a selective thoracic fusion. The definition of selective fusion is when both MT and TL/L deviate completely from the midline, but only the major curve is fused and the minor curve is left unfused and mobile.[5] Importantly, for the TL/L curves the midline means the central sacral vertical line (CSVL), whereas for MT curves the midline is the C7 plumb line (C7PL) (**Fig. 6.2**). The aim of performing a selective fusion is to spare motion segments, which is the most challenging decision in the surgical treatment of AIS. To help with this difficult

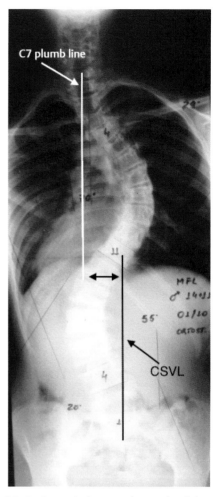

Fig. 6.2 Radiograph showing the C7 plumb line and central sacral vertical line (CSVL). The trunk shift is the distance between the lines.

decision, Lenke et al described clinical and radiographic criteria (see **Box 6.1**).[5] Even if all the criteria above are met, a selective fusion should be avoided in patients with a trunk shift to the left of more than 2 cm (C7PL – CSVL > 2 cm), due to the high risk of postoperative imbalance.[9]

If a selective fusion is recommended, then the LIV should be the SV.[10] When it is not possible to perform a selective fusion, the lumbar curve must be included in the arthrodesis, and selecting the LIV follows the same rules for the lumbar curves, as we shall see in the next subsection.

Box 6.1 Radiographic and Clinical Criteria for Selective Thoracic Fusion

Radiographic Criteria
- MT:TL/L Ratio > 1.2 (Cobb, AVT, AVR)
- TL/L more flexible than MT (ideally < 25 degrees on bending film)
- Absence of thoracolumbar transitional kyphosis over 10 degrees (T10–L2 < 10 degrees)

Clinical Criteria
- Patient with the right shoulder higher or both shoulders level
- Thoracic trunk shift more pronounced than the waistline asymmetry
- Thoracic scoliometer measurement greater then the lumbar scoliometer measurement with at least a 1.2 ratio

Abbreviations: MT, main thoracic curve; TL/L, thoracolumbar/lumbar curve; AVT, apical vertebral translation; AVR, apical vertebral rotation.

Step 4: Choosing the Upper Instrumented Vertebra for Thoracolumbar/Lumbar Curves (Lenke 5 and 6)

The selection of the UIV depends on whether the thoracic curve is to be included or not. In Lenke 5 curves, it usually is not necessary to include the MT, and the UIV should be the PEV.[11,12] However, the MT needs to be included in some patients, especially in those with a clinically evident thoracic rib hump or with a right shoulder higher than the left. This is because the right shoulder tends to become higher and the thoracic rib hump tends to become more evident postoperatively. In Lenke 6C curves, deciding whether or not to perform a selective fusion is usually more difficult. To make this decision, the clinical and radiographic criteria are very similar to those utilized in the major MT with lumbar modifier type C (see **Box 6.2**). This is an important point to be discussed with the patient and family before surgery.

For a selective fusion, the UIV is usually the PEV of the lumbar curve.[11,12] If there are no conditions for a selective lumbar fusion, the UIV is chosen as the major MT in which PT does not need to be included, generally stopping at NV.

Step 5: Choosing the Lower Instrumented Vertebra for Thoracolumbar/Lumbar Curves (Lenke 5 and 6)

The LIV is usually L3 or L4. According to Shuflebarger et al,[11] the LIV should be the DEV.[12] Suk et al[4,8] divided the TL/L into types A and B. In type A, the L3 crosses the CSVL on the bending X-rays, and the rotation of L3 is less than grade 2. In these cases, the LIV may be L3. When the L3 rotation is greater than grade 2 or does not cross the CSVL on the bending films, the LIV should be L4.[4,8] Nevertheless, in practice, both rules are usually concordant.

▦ Role of Anterior Surgery

The anterior approach for idiopathic scoliosis is selected for the following indications:

The Same Access for Correction and Definitive Instrumentation

The anterior instrumentation of the spine in AIS is indicated only for deformities with a single structured curve (Lenke 1 or 5). It may be performed by a thoracoscopic approach in the thoracic spine (Lenke 1).[13] It is contraindicated in overweight patients (> 70 kg) or in the presence of hyperkyphosis, rigid curves (< 25% of correction on bending films), and curves > 70 degrees.[14] The fusion levels should include all the curvature (PEV to DEV). Currently, the anterior approach has not been widely used for many reasons: restricted indications; the difficulty of dealing with complications such as pseudarthrosis or instrumentation failure, which usually require a complementary surgery from the back; and the long learning curve for the thoracoscopic approach with instrumentation. Moreover, some studies show similar or better results with the posterior

---

Box 6.2 Radiographic and Clinical Criteria for Selective TL/L Fusion

Radiographic Criteria
- TL/L:MT Ratio > 1.25 (Cobb, AVT, AVR)
- MT more flexible than TL/L (ideally < 25 degrees on bending film)
- Absence of thoracolumbar transitional kyphosis over 20 degrees (T10–L2 < 20 degrees)

Clinical Criteria
- Patient with the left shoulder higher or both shoulders level
- Waistline asymmetry more pronounced than thoracic trunk shift
- Lumbar scoliometer measurement greater than thoracic scoliometer measurement with at least a 1.2 ratio
- Thoracic cage deformity acceptable to patient and family and to surgeon preoperatively

Source: Adapted from Lenke LG, Edwards II CC, Bridwell KH. The Lenke classification of adolescent idiopathic scoliosis: how to organizes curve patterns as a template to perform selective of the spine. Spine 2003; 28:S199–S207.

approach, which is the most familiar one to spine surgeons.[13,15]

As a First Stage to Anterior Release, Followed by Posterior Instrumentation and Fusion

With the advent of pedicle screws and the development of many release and shortening techniques using the posterior-only approach (Ponte's osteotomy, Smith-Petersen osteotomy, pedicle subtraction osteotomy, posterior vertebral column resection), the anterior approach is no longer needed to make rigid curves (> 70 degrees) more flexible,[13] thus avoiding the violation of the ribcage that may impair the pulmonary function. Nonetheless, surgeons who do not have intraoperative neuromonitoring available or who are not familiar with these posterior osteotomies may still use it. The goals are to release the curve, which permits more correction from the subsequent posterior approach, and to decrease the risks of pseudarthrosis and neurologic injury.

To Prevent the Crankshaft Phenomenon in Immature Patients[16]

The anterior approach may also be used to avoid the crankshaft phenomenon in very young children, especially when the triradiate cartilage is still open at the moment of definitive arthrodesis,[17,18] and to halt anterior spinal growth by circumferential fusion. However, it has been suggested that pedicle screws have the capacity of controlling the vertebrae anteriorly, which reduces the risk of developing the crankshaft phenomenon, and making the anterior fusion unnecessary to prevent anterior growing in these very young children.[19]

In Patients with Remarkable Thoracic Hypokyphosis

Although hypokyphosis is frequent in AIS patients, a true thoracic lordosis is very uncommon. In fact, for these rare cases, the anterior approach to the spine in AIS is currently the best indication. The anterior approach enables the anterior shortening of the spine and permits the restoration of kyphosis in the thoracic spine,[13] but in most AIS patients with hypokyphosis, adequate sagittal alignment can be restored using multiple Ponte's osteotomies associated with more rigid rods, such as chromo-cobalt or stainless steel rods.

Chapter Summary

After the development of the modern pedicle screw instrumentation and the development of the Lenke classification system,[2,3] it has been possible to predict the postoperative behavior of different AIS curves. A precise and methodical clinical and radiographic evaluation is required to select the correct fusion levels in AIS patients. The decision-making process of determining the UIV and LIV have been presented. The selection of the fusion levels is fundamental in achieving the goals of AIS treatment and obtaining a tridimensional realignment spine while preserving as many levels as possible.

Pearls

I. Classify the deformity with the Lenke classification system[3] and identify the SV and NV.
II. Thoracic curves
   A. UIV: include the PT?
     1. Yes: T2
     2. No: proximal NV
   B. LIV
     1. Structured TL/L: lumbar DEV
     2. Nonstructured TL/L
       a. Lumbar modifier AL or B: SV
       b. Lumbar modifier AR: NV or NV-1
       c. Lumbar modifier C: selective fusion?
         i. Yes: SV
         ii. No: lumbar DEV
III. TL/L curves: selective fusion?
   A. Yes: PEV to DEV
   B. No: Proximal thoracic NV to DEV

Pitfalls

- Inadequate positioning of the patient when taking X-rays (proper positioning: hands on shoulder, extended knees).
- Inadequate attention to structural regional factors (T2–T5 and T10–L2 regional kyphosis).[3]
- Lack of care when performing selective fusion in immature patients. Avoid fusing patients with the triradiate cartilage open because of the risk of proximal adding on, crankshaft phenomenon, and less correction of the lumbar C curves.[20]

- Failure to use a good arthrodesis technique to obtain a solid fusion.
- Failure to consider the physical exam when determining the fusion levels, especially the shoulder levels, trunk balance, and rotational deformity.
- A thoracic selective posterior arthrodesis in patients unbalanced preoperatively greatly increases the risk of maintaining this imbalance postoperatively.[9] Thoracic selective posterior arthrodesis should be avoided in these patients.

References

Five Must-Read References

1. King HA, Moe JH, Bradford DS, Winter RB. The selection of fusion levels in thoracic idiopathic scoliosis. J Bone Joint Surg Am 1983;65:1302–1313

2. Lenke LG, Betz RR, Harms J, et al. Adolescent idiopathic scoliosis: a new classification to determine extent of spinal arthrodesis. J Bone Joint Surg Am 2001;83-A:1169–1181

3. Kim HJ, de Kleuver M, Luk K. Online reference in clinical life: Deformity. AO Surgery Reference. https://www2.aofoundation.org/wps/portal/surgery?showPage=diagnosis&bone=Spine&segment=Deformity Published July 2013; accessed May 2016

4. Suk SI, Kim JH, Kim SS, Lim DJ. Pedicle screw instrumentation in adolescent idiopathic scoliosis (AIS). Eur Spine J 2012;21:13–22

5. Lenke LG, Edwards CC II, Bridwell KH. The Lenke classification of adolescent idiopathic scoliosis: how it organizes curve patterns as a template to perform selective fusions of the spine. Spine 2003;28:S199–S207

6. Lenke LG, Bridwell KH, O'Brien MF, Baldus C, Blanke K. Recognition and treatment of the proximal thoracic curve in adolescent idiopathic scoliosis treated with Cotrel-Dubousset instrumentation. Spine 1994; 19:1589–1597

7. Miyanji F, Pawelek JB, Van Valin SE, Upasani VV, Newton PO. Is the lumbar modifier useful in surgical decision making?: defining two distinct Lenke 1A curve patterns. Spine 2008;33:2545–2551

8. Suk SI, Lee SM, Chung ER, Kim JHK, Kim WJ, Sohn HM. Determination of distal fusion level with segmental pedicle screw fixation in single thoracic idiopathic scoliosis. Spine 2003;28:484–491

9. Demura S, Yaszay B, Bastrom TP, Carreau J, Newton PO; Harms Study Group. Is decompensation preoperatively a risk in Lenke 1C curves? Spine 2013;38: E649–E655

10. Trobisch PD, Ducoffe AR, Lonner BS, Errico TJ. Choosing fusion levels in adolescent idiopathic scoliosis. J Am Acad Orthop Surg 2013;21:519–528

11. Shufflebarger HL, Geck MJ, Clark CE. The posterior approach for lumbar and thoracolumbar adolescent idiopathic scoliosis: posterior shortening and pedicle screws. Spine 2004;29:269–276, discussion 276

12. Geck MJ, Rinella A, Hawthorne D, et al. Anterior dual rod versus pedicle fixation for the surgical treatment in Lenke 5C adolescent idiopathic scoliosis: a multicenter, matched case analysis of 42 patients. Spine Deform 2013;1:217–222

13. Newton PO, Upasani VV. Surgical treatment of the right thoracic curve pattern. In: Newton PO, O'Brien MF, Shufflebarger HL, et al, eds. Idiopathic Scoliosis: The Harms Study Group Treatment Guide. New York: Thieme; 2010:200–223

14. Letko L, Jensen RG, Harms J. The treatment of rigid adolescent idiopathic scoliosis: releases, osteotomies, and apical vertebral column resection. In: Newton PO, O'Brien MF, Shufflebarger HL, et al, eds. Idiopathic Scoliosis: The Harms Study Group Treatment Guide. New York: Thieme; 2010:188–199

15. Geck MJ, Rinella A, Hawthorne D, et al. Comparison of surgical treatment in Lenke 5C adolescent idiopathic scoliosis: anterior dual rod versus posterior pedicle fixation surgery: a comparison of two practices. Spine 2009;34:1942–1951

16. Dubousset J, Herring JA, Shufflebarger H. The crankshaft phenomenon. J Pediatr Orthop 1989;9:541–550

17. Lapinksy AS, Richards BS. Preventing the crankshaft phenomenon by combining anterior fusion with posterior instrumentation. Does it work? Spine 1995; 20:1392–1398

18. Shufflebarger HL, Clark CE. Prevention of the crankshaft phenomenon. Spine 1991; 16(8, Suppl):S409–S411

19. Suk SI, Kim JH, Cho KJ, Kim SS, Lee JJ, Han YT. Is anterior release necessary in severe scoliosis treated by posterior segmental pedicle screw fixation? Eur Spine J 2007;16:1359–1365

20. Sponseller PD, Betz R, Newton PO, et al; Harms Study Group. Differences in curve behavior after fusion in adolescent idiopathic scoliosis patients with open tri-radiate cartilages. Spine 2009;34:827–831.

7

Novel Nonfusion Growth-Modulating Techniques for Pediatric Scoliosis

Caglar Yilgor and Ahmet Alanay

Introduction

It is well understood that curve correction in the growing child's spine does not always result in a healthy child due to the potentially life-threatening long-term side effects of early spinal fusion. Definitive fusion in a growing spine retards or halts longitudinal spinal growth, spinal canal formation, thoracic cage growth, and lung development. This results in a disproportionately short trunk, possible crankshafting and adding on, and respiratory insufficiency.

As the drawbacks of early fusion were better understood, the concept of "delaying tactics" was suggested.[1] These nonoperative and operative tactics aim to delay fusion for as long as possible, if not to totally avoid it. Nonoperative delaying tactics include traction, casting, and bracing. Operative delaying tactics intend to control the deformity while allowing growth of the spine, thoracic cage, and lungs.[2]

Growth-modulating procedures such as vertebral body stapling and tethering may provide substantial advantages over both nonoperative and operative delaying tactics, and may lead to definitive spinal fusion in a selected group of patients. The purpose of growth-modulating methods is to harness the patient's inherent spinal growth and redirect it to achieve correction, rather than progression, of the curve.[3]

This is accomplished by applying compressive forces on convexity via an anterior approach.

Overview of Nonfusion Techniques

Nonfusion surgical techniques are employed to achieve deformity correction; to allow spinal, thoracic cage, and thus lung growth; to maintain correction during the growth period; and to postpone or avoid fusion. The most commonly used nonfusion techniques can be grouped in four categories (**Table 7.1**). Growth preservation/stimulation, growth guidance, and growth modulation are the three main surgical philosophies. Combinations of these techniques with or without limited fusion are referred to as the fourth category of hybrid constructs. Growth modulation is discussed in detail later in this chapter. Detailed information on other growth-sparing techniques can be found in Chapter 5.

Growth preservation and stimulation techniques are distraction-based constructs in which a mobile spinal segment exists with anchor foundations at either end. They are named based on the location and type of the foundations. Regular lengthenings are applied to control or correct the curves while preserving and

Table 7.1 Nonfusion Surgical Techniques Commonly Used for Early-Onset and Immature Adolescent Idiopathic Scoliosis

Growth preservation/stimulation	Posterior spinal distraction • Single growing rod • Dual growing rod • Magnetically controlled growing rod intercostal/costovertebral distractions • Expansion thoracoplasty • Vertical, expandable prosthetic titanium rib
Growth guidance	• Shilla technique • Modern Luque trolley • Sliding growing rod
Growth modulation	• Vertebral body stapling • Vertebral body tethering
Hybrid constructs and others	• Convex growth arrest + concave distraction • Limited fusion + growth stimulation • Distraction-aided growth guidance • Fusionless, multiple vertebral wedge osteotomies

possibly reinforcing the spinal growth due to the effect of distraction on immature vertebral growth.[4,5] But observations of spinal fibrosis, ankylosis, and autofusion led to criticism of such techniques.[6,7] Additionally, these constructs were associated with numerous planned and unplanned reoperations with a high rate of complications, including anchor dislodgment or rod breakages, wound problems, and alignment issues.[8] Although the ideal has probably not yet been reached, more recently available magnetically controlled growing rods can be lengthened noninvasively, reducing the number of repetitive surgeries.[8]

Growth guidance techniques include apical control to achieve a better correction and lessen the transitional stresses on the unfused spine while abandoning the effect of the use of distractive forces. These self-sliding assemblies preclude the need for many additional procedures and provide adequate maintenance of curve correction in most cases, although the spinal growth obtained may be less than expected.[9]

Hybrid constructs may include convex growth arrest plus concave distraction,[10] limited fusion plus growing rods, and distraction-aided growth guidance. Maruyama et al[11] defined a fusionless procedure of noninstrumented multiple vertebral wedge osteotomies via open thoracotomy as a definitive surgical treatment of immature and mature adolescent idiopathic scoliosis (AIS).

Growth Modulation for Pediatric Scoliosis

Treatment options for skeletally immature idiopathic scoliosis patients with moderate curves have long been limited to observation and bracing.[12,13] Observation resulted in spinal fusion in 75% of pubertal onset curves between 21 and 30 degrees and 100% of curves > 30 degrees at the onset of puberty.[14] Observation entails taking periodic radiographs, and the patient and family can experience anxiety associated with the possibility of progression.

Bracing has therefore remained the standard of care, although clinical results widely varied. The recent Bracing in Adolescent Idiopathic Scoliosis Trial (BrAIST) found that appropriately prepared and worn braces reduced the need for surgical treatment by 50%.[13] Nevertheless, brace wear requires the child's commitment for 16 to 23 hours per day. The brace is cumbersome and uncomfortable, especially in warm climates and during the summer. Brace treatment typically requires 3 to 5 years, and possibly even longer depending on when the child starts wearing one. As bracing requires significant compliance and can have social implications, the potential success of this treatment modality can be compromised. Furthermore, some patients experience psychosocial stress regarding their body image; they feel that their body asymmetry is worse than that of untreated scoliosis patients, despite similar curve sizes.[15,16]

In a logical sense, patients bear the cumbersome bracing treatment not to avoid surgery but to avoid spinal fusion, which, to date, remains the most viable surgical option in scoliosis treatment. Yet fusion entails decreased spinal mobility, decreased range of motion, inhibition of growth over the length of the construct, and the possible development of adjacent segment degeneration.[17–19]

Thus, growth- and motion-sparing strategies that modulate the growth of the spine, stabilize the curve, and avoid spinal fusion are alternatives to bracing for the treatment of progressive scoliosis. These growth-modulating techniques address the remaining spinal growth of the child and are generally referred to as tension-based or convexity compression methods. The logic behind applying compression to the convexity of the curve is based on the Hueter-Volkmann law that states that a growth plate under pressure will grow more slowly than one that is subjected to less pressure.[20]

Vertebral Body Stapling

Vertebral body stapling is an alternative to bracing for the treatment of progressive scoliosis in late juvenile and immature AIS.

Interestingly, vertebral stapling originated in the 1950s, when wire staples were placed across the disk spaces. The Hueter-Volkmann principle was first tested in canines[21] and then applied in three humans.[22] When this attempt was unsuccessful due to implant migration, the procedure was abandoned until recently.

Implant design with shape-memory metals and use of video-assisted thoracoscopy have breathed new life into this procedure.[23] Nitinol (an acronym for the former *Ni*ckel *Ti*tanium

*Na*val *O*rdnance *L*aboratory, White Oak, MD, where it was developed) is a biocompatible shape-memory metal alloy that is implanted in a cooled state. The prongs of the staple are perpendicular. Once the metal warms to body temperature, the prongs clamp down on the end plate, providing a gentle compressive force and diminishing the risk of pullout.[24]

Surgical Technique

For thoracic curves, the child is placed in the lateral decubitus position, with the curve convexity facing up.[25] To enable slight correction of the curve, an axillary roll is placed underneath the concave side. Video-assisted thoracoscopy is used with single lung ventilation and carbon dioxide insufflation. Vertebral bodies are identified using biplanar fluoroscopy. Staples are first placed in ice.

The instrumentation is performed from end to end vertebrae. Care is taken to protect the segmental vessels because they are located in the middle of the body and not in the implantation site. A trial is used at every level to gauge the size. To help with the correction, the trial device can be used to push on the apex. Then the trial is removed and the staple is quickly inserted. Optimal staple placement requires that the prongs be close to the vertebral end plate.[25] The staple is placed anterior to the rib head in the sagittal plane. A more anterior position is desired in hypokyphotic curves. After the optimal position of the staple is fluoroscopically confirmed, the staple is impacted in the vertebral body. These steps are repeated at every level. At the end of the procedure, a chest tube drain is placed.[25]

For lumbar curves, a direct lateral, retroperitoneal approach with a minimal open incision[26] is preferred.[25] The psoas muscle is retracted posteriorly or is separated longitudinally over the posterior half of the disk under electromyographic control. Staples are placed at three or four levels in the posterior half of the vertebral body.[25]

It is important to maximize the intraoperative correction, because results are more favorable when curves are reduced to < 20 degrees in the first standing radiographs.[25]

Results

Vertebral body stapling works by slowing the growth of the convexity of the curve using the same principle as hemiepiphysiodesis. Shape memory staples compress and bridge the growth plates to reversibly reduce or block growth. In theory, implants avoid the need for definitive asymmetric spinal fusion. Yet there are concerns regarding stiffening of the instrumented segments[27] that may lead to disk degeneration or spontaneous fusion. Betz et al[24] demonstrated the feasibility, safety, and utility of this technique in immature AIS.

To better interpret the results, thoracic and lumbar curves should be analyzed separately because they respond differently to stapling. Betz et al[28] reported results for stapling of 52 curves in 39 patients of ages 8 years and older, in whom progression was ≤ 10 degrees in 87% of the patients at a minimum 1-year follow-up. Longer follow-up revealed similar results of ≤ 10 degrees progression of ~ 78% in all lumbar curves and thoracic curves < 35 degrees.[25]

Later, the same group compared the results of stapling versus bracing in moderate scoliotic patients with a high-risk of progression.[29] The success rate for 25- to 34-degree thoracic curves was 81%, versus 61% for stapling and bracing. For larger thoracic curves measuring 35 to 44 degrees the treatment success rate was 18% versus 50% for stapling and bracing. For lumbar curves of 25 to 34 degrees, the success rates for stapling and for bracing were similar, 80% and 81%; for larger lumbar curves, however, these success rates were 60% and 0%. Nonetheless, it is difficult to draw any conclusions for > 35-degree lumbar curves, because only five patients underwent stapling, and only two were braced.[29]

Poor results were consistently reported in thoracic curves > 35 degrees.[25,28,29] In these curves, the general mode of failure was that the instrumented curve remained stable, but the curvature increased at the two ends of the construct,[30] subsequently necessitating fusion. In contrast, in a series of 12 children younger than 10 years of age with thoracic and lumbar scoliosis of 30 to 39 degrees, vertebral body stapling was found to be effective, as the children either had no change in their curve or had curve improvement.[31]

Complications associated with stapling, although infrequent, include dislodged or broken staples, curve overcorrection, pneumothorax, congenital diaphragmatic hernia rupture, contralateral pleural effusion, and superior mesenteric artery syndrome.[25,29,32,33]

Indications

It is difficult to determine when an operative intervention should be applied to patients who currently are being offered nonoperative treatment with either observation or a brace.[25] Better stratification of curve progression risks may help identify high-risk patients who are stapling candidates.

Based on the current literature, the recommended indications for vertebral body stapling are as follows[29]: (1) age < 13 years in girls and < 15 years in boys; (2) Sanders score[34] < 5; (3) thoracic curves ≤ 35 degrees and lumbar coronal curves ≤ 45 degrees; and (4) sagittal thoracic kyphosis < 40 degrees. However, the use of these implants for this indication is not yet approved by the Food and Drug Administration (FDA).

If the curve does not measure < 20 degrees after stapling on the first standing radiograph, then it is recommended that the patient wear a corrective brace at nighttime until it does or until skeletal maturity is reached.[25] If the thoracic curve measures 35 to 45 degrees or does not bend below 20 degrees even for curves < 35 degrees, then vertebral body tethering should be considered instead of stapling.[29]

There is limited Level 4 (case series) evidence that well-selected pediatric scoliosis patients with significant growth potential and moderate curves can be safely treated with vertebral body stapling as an alternative to bracing (**Fig. 7.1**).

▌ Vertebral Body Tethering

Vertebral body tethering is the application of vertebral body screws on the convexity and the

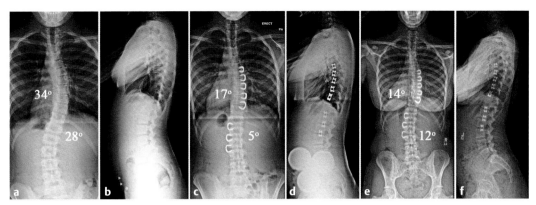

Fig. 7.1 An 11-year-old girl who had a progressive 34-degree thoracic/28-degree lumbar curvature. She was Risser grade 0 and progressed despite bracing. She underwent vertebral body stapling of T5 to T11 and lumbar tethering of T12 to L3. **(a,b)** Preoperative radiographs. **(c,d)** Postoperatively, she appeared to be well balanced. **(e,f)** Five years postoperatively, she has maintained her correction. (Courtesy of Amer Samdani.)

attachment of a polyethylene tether that is then shortened and tightened. It is indicated for immature AIS through a minimally invasive thoracoscopic access to the anterior thoracic spine. The remaining growth potential of the child will urge more growth on the concavity, thereby lessening or reversing the deformity.

The biomechanical basis for tethering was first demonstrated in porcine[35] and goat[36] models. Staples and tethers were compared in the goat model.[37] The results demonstrated greater efficacy and integrity with tethers compared with the more rigid shape-memory alloy staples. The tether provided an increased flexibility that decreased the forces during spinal motion and protected the bone anchors from loosening. A halo was observed around the prongs of the staples, whereas the vertebral body screws of the tether provided better fixation to the bone.[37] This increased flexibility possibly contributed to greater mobility and as a consequence, a lower risk of spontaneous fusion.[38]

Surgical Technique

Patient positioning and the thoracoscopy setup is similar to that for stapling. For tethering, the pleura is dissected off the lateral aspect of the vertebral bodies anterior to the rib heads sequentially along the length of the curve.[39] Segmental vessels are identified, coagulated, and divided because the implantation will be at the midcorpus level. Care is taken to protect the intervertebral disks.

The instrumentation is performed from the end to end vertebrae. Either the screws can be directly placed, or a three-prong staple may be used to facilitate insertion and stabilization. The screws are inserted anterior to the rib head and directed toward the concavity across the anterolateral aspect of the vertebral body. In this manner, the screws are sequentially placed from cephalad to caudal moving the access port into the next lower intercostal space through the same skin incision. Instrumentation can be done via this approach down to L1 or L2. Instrumentation to L3 (and occasionally L2) requires a mini-open retroperitoneal approach.

The tether is then passed up through the caudal port and placed within the tulips of the screws. The set screws on each screw are tightened one by one while achieving correction through both tensioning of the tether and translation of the spine. The residual tether is cut, leaving at least 2 cm at either end to accommodate potential future tether adjustment. At the end of the procedure, a chest tube drain is placed. A protective brace is suggested to be worn for 4 to 6 weeks.

Thoracoscopic anterior vertebral body tethering can be combined with a lumbar stapling procedure.

Results

After the promising results from animal studies, the first reported human case was an 8.5-year-old patient with a 40-degree thoracic curve. The curve was reduced to 25 degrees in the first postoperative standing radiograph, and, with further growth, progressively corrected down to 8 degrees over 48 months.[40] A series of 32 patients similarly demonstrated a progressive correction of their major coronal Cobb angle at 1-year follow-up.[39] Rib prominence also improved ~ 50%, likely due to the coupled motion of the spine in different planes where correcting one plane results in some improvement in the others.[41]

Later, other larger cohort reports demonstrated results similar to those of the first reported case.[39,42] Overall, the results look promising, with additional time- and growth-dependent correction attained after initial surgery. There is even the possibility of overcorrection and of reversing of the curve in 10

to 15% of patients. This may require a repeat thoracoscopic approach to loosen the tether.

In recent studies, 1-year[39] and 2-year[42] follow-up results showed a stable or improved coronal Cobb angle, thoracic scoliometer reading, and coronal balance. The main thoracic and compensatory lumbar curves displayed additional correction in the course of follow-up, whereas proximal thoracic curves remained stable after the initial correction.

Additional correction attained during follow-up is time and growth dependent. For main thoracic curves, 12.5% of the patients were reported to achieve more than 10 degrees of correction. Some were overcorrected, resulting in reversed curves to negative Cobb angles. It was found that 28% of the patients attained between 5 and 10 degrees of correction, and 56% remained stable, measuring within 5 degrees of the first erect radiograph; 3% had a slight loss of correction over time.[39]

Mean early postoperative thoracic kyphosis and lumbar lordosis showed a slight decrease after surgery, but returned to the initial values during follow-up[39,42] (**Fig. 7.2**).

Rotational correction measured with the scoliometer was about 40%; 88% of the patients

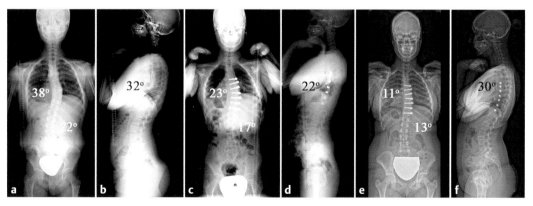

Fig. 7.2 An 11-year-old girl presented to our clinic with a 38-degree right thoracic curve and a 22-degree left lumbar curve. Thoracic kyphosis was 32 degrees. **(a)** Preoperative anteroposterior (AP) and **(b)** lateral radiographs of the patient undergoing anterior vertebral body tethering. (She was our first case.) **(c)** First postoperative standing AP and **(d)** lateral radiographs after thoracoscopic anterior vertebral body tethering show that the thoracic curve corrected to 23 degrees and the lumbar curve to 17 degrees. Thoracic kyphosis was 22 degrees. At age 13, which was 24 months postoperative, the thoracic curve measures 11 degrees and the lumbar 13 degrees on the AP radiograph **(e),** and the thoracic kyphosis measures 30 degrees on the lateral radiograph **(f)**. The patient is Risser grade 5.

had ≥ 10 degrees rib prominence preoperatively, whereas only 28% and 18% had a measurement > 10 degrees at 1- and 2-year follow-up, respectively.[39,42]

Overall coronal and sagittal balance remained stable with a statistically insignificant improvement in coronal balance.[42] Shoulder balance did not significantly change. To date, all reported patients have not needed a spinal fusion and have subjectively retained spinal mobility. Operative time and estimated blood loss had a marked decrease as surgical experience accumulated.[42]

No neurologic, infectious, or implant-related complications were reported.[39,42] Persistent atelectasis can require bronchoscopy. Worsening of the deformity can occur but is not likely, and there is always the possibility of correction as long as the child has some remaining growth potential (**Fig. 7.3**). Overcorrection is anticipated especially for younger children with Risser grade 0. As surgical experience is gained, the ability to judge the amount of correction to impart during the initial surgery is improving, which should decrease the chances of overcorrection.[39]

Indications

Although similar in theory to the technique of vertebral body stapling, tethering has the theoretical advantage of applying more acute corrective translational and compressive forces onto the curve during placement. Therefore, it may be indicated for larger curves (> 35 degrees) where stapling has proven to be ineffective.

Current indications for this technique include the following: (1) skeletally immature patients with idiopathic scoliosis and curves between 35 and 60 degrees; (2) at least 50% flexibility or bending to < 30 degrees; (3) thoracic kyphosis of < 40 degrees; and (4) rotational prominence < 20 degrees. Skeletal maturity is determined using a variety of factors including the Risser sign ≤ 2, Sanders score ≤ 4, and menarche status.[42] However, the use of these implants for this indication is not yet approved by the FDA.

Although the use of tethering for more severe scoliosis is yet to be demonstrated, family history, parental height, child's height, secondary sex characteristics, and other factors may also influence the use of these general indications.[42] For instance, tethering may

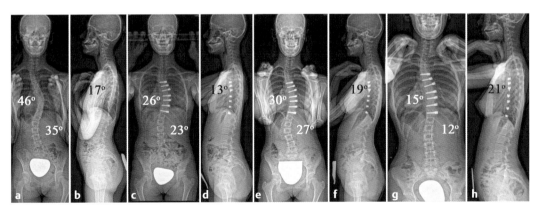

Fig. 7.3 An 11-year-old girl presented to our clinic with a 46-degree right thoracic curve and a 35-degree left lumbar curve. Thoracic kyphosis was 17 degrees. (**a**) Preoperative AP and (**b**) lateral radiographs. (**c**) First postoperative standing AP and (**d**) lateral radiographs after thoracoscopic anterior vertebral body tethering show that the thoracic curve corrected to 26 degrees and the lumbar curve to 23 degrees. Thoracic kyphosis was 13 degrees. (**e**) Four months postoperative radiographs displayed progression of both curves. The thoracic curve measured 30 degrees and the lumbar curve measured 27 degrees. (**f**) Thoracic kyphosis improved to 13 degrees. At age 12, which was 12 postoperative, the thoracic curve measures 15 degrees and the lumbar 12 degrees on the AP radiograph (**g**), and thoracic kyphosis measures 21 degrees on the lateral radiograph (**h**). The patient is Risser grade 2.

be considered for a curve > 60 degrees as long as it bends to less than 30 degrees. Yet the upper limits for thoracic kyphosis and rotation are absolute. Although restoration of thoracic kyphosis is one of the surgical goals of scoliosis surgery,[43,44] excessive kyphosis is not desirable. To limit the potential hyperkyphosing effects of anterior surgery, a thoracic kyphosis of > 40 degrees is considered a contraindication. Although placing the apical screws slightly more posteriorly may encourage additional derotation, vertebral body tethering is not recommended for a child with a > 20 degrees of rib prominence, as it is unlikely to attain sufficient correction.[39]

Generally, the ideal candidate is a child who is 10 years of age or older, although application in patients as young as 8.5 years has been reported.[40] The rationale behind this age threshold is that the current instrumentation is not accommodated in younger children with smaller vertebral bodies, and that this powerful technique can lead to overcorrection. The use of anterior vertebral body tethering in children younger than 8 years of age is therefore not recommended, because evidence is lacking that spinal growth will return to normal once the tether is cut after the manifestation of overcorrection.[8]

In general, vertebral body tethering is a safe and efficient procedure that may provide substantial advantages over both nonoperative and operative delaying tactics, and definitive spinal fusion in a selected group of patients.

Chapter Summary and Future Directions

This is a time of great changes in spine surgery. In an environment of changing health care ethics and reimbursement necessities, technology is rapidly developing with many promising treatments. Patients are becoming more educated about their diagnoses, treatment options, and outcomes than ever before. Minimally invasive surgery techniques, growth-sparing and motion-preserving applications, and micro-electronics that can monitor and respond to changing conditions hold promise for further development.

Growth modulation with anterior convexity vertebral body compression is a promising alternative to bracing and fusion surgery for pediatric scoliosis. Although the indications are limited today, growth modulation is a promising technique to avoid fusion and related consequences. It is important to obtain longer term follow-up to demonstrate the true benefit of this technique. Modifications to adopt this nonfusion technique for applicability in even younger children and late adolescents will be revolutionary. This may allow a permanent solution for scoliosis with one nonfusion surgery.

Today, many steps have been taken in not fusing the spinal column. The future of spine medicine may totally avoid surgery by applying a form of external inhibitor (such as a wave or beam) noninvasively to limit the growth of the convex side of the vertebral growth plates, or even to stimulate the concavity. The ultimate aim is to reveal the etiology of scoliosis to prevent it totally.

Pearls

- The recommended indications for vertebral body stapling are as follows: (1) age < 13 years in girls and < 15 years in boys; (2) Sanders score < 5; (3) thoracic curves ≤ 35 degrees and lumbar coronal curves ≤ 45 degrees; and (4) sagittal thoracic curve <40 degrees.
- It is important to maximize the intraoperative correction with stapling, because results are more favorable when the thoracic curves are reduced to < 20 degrees in the first standing radiographs.
- If the curve does not measure < 20 degrees after stapling on the first standing radiograph, it is recommended that the patient wear a corrective brace at nighttime until it does or until skeletal maturity is reached.
- If the thoracic curve measures 35 to 45 degrees or does not bend below 20 degrees even for curves < 35 degrees, vertebral body tethering should be considered instead of stapling.

◆ Current indications for this anterior vertebral body tethering include the following: (1) skeletally immature patients with idiopathic scoliosis and curves between 35 and 60 degrees; (2) at least 50% flexibility or bending to < 30 degrees; (3) thoracic kyphosis of < 40 degrees; and (4) rotational prominence < 20 degrees.

◆ It is important to judge the amount of correction to impart during the initial surgery to decrease the risk of overcorrection.

Pitfalls

◆ To limit the potential hyperkyphosing effects of anterior surgery, a thoracic kyphosis of > 40 degrees is considered a contraindication for vertebral body stapling and tethering.

◆ Vertebral body stapling and tethering is not recommended for a child with a > 20 degrees of rib prominence measured with the inclinometer as it is unlikely to obtain sufficient correction.

References

Five Must-Read References

1. Johnston CE. Delaying tactics: traction, casting and bracing. In: Yazici M, ed. Non-idiopathic Spine Deformities in Young Children. Heidelberg: New York: Springer; 2011:109–121

2. Akbarnia BA. Management themes in early onset scoliosis. J Bone Joint Surg Am 2007;89(Suppl 1):42–54

3. Guille JT, D'Andrea LP, Betz RR. Fusionless treatment of scoliosis. Orthop Clin North Am 2007;38:541–545, vii

4. Olgun ZD, Ahmadiadli H, Alanay A, Yazici M. Vertebral body growth during growing rod instrumentation: growth preservation or stimulation? J Pediatr Orthop 2012;32:184–189

5. Yilmaz G, Huri G, Demirkran G, et al. The effect of posterior distraction on vertebral growth in immature pigs: an experimental simulation of growing rod technique. Spine 2010;35:730–733

6. Cahill PJ, Marvil S, Cuddihy L, et al. Autofusion in the immature spine treated with growing rods. Spine 2010;35:E1199–E1203

7. Flynn JM, Tomlinson LA, Pawelek J, Thompson GH, McCarthy R, Akbarnia BA; Growing Spine Study Group. Growing-rod graduates: lessons learned from ninety-nine patients who completed lengthening. J Bone Joint Surg Am 2013;95:1745–1750

8. Cunin V. Early-onset scoliosis: current treatment. Orthop Traumatol Surg Res 2015;101(1, Suppl):S109–S118

9. Odent T, Ilharreborde B, Miladi L, et al; Scoliosis Study Group (Groupe d'étude de la scoliose); French Society of Pediatric Orthopedics (SOFOP). Fusionless surgery in early-onset scoliosis. Orthop Traumatol Surg Res 2015;101(6, Suppl):S281–S288

10. Alanay A, Dede O, Yazici M. Convex instrumented hemiepiphysiodesis with concave distraction: a preliminary report. Clin Orthop Relat Res 2012;470:1144–1150

11. Maruyama T, Kitagawa T, Takeshita K, et al. Fusionless surgery for scoliosis: 2–17 year radiographic and clinical follow-up. Spine 2006;31:2310–2315

12. Nachemson AL, Peterson LE. Effectiveness of treatment with a brace in girls who have adolescent idiopathic scoliosis. A prospective, controlled study based on data from the Brace Study of the Scoliosis Research Society. J Bone Joint Surg Am 1995;77:815–822

13. Weinstein SL, Dolan LA, Wright JG, Dobbs MB. Effects of bracing in adolescents with idiopathic scoliosis. N Engl J Med 2013;369:1512–1521

14. Charles YP, Daures JP, de Rosa V, Diméglio A. Progression risk of idiopathic juvenile scoliosis during pubertal growth. Spine 2006;31:1933–1942

15. Fällström K, Cochran T, Nachemson A. Long-term effects on personality development in patients with adolescent idiopathic scoliosis. Influence of type of treatment. Spine 1986;11:756–758

16. Misterska E, Glowacki M, Latuszewska J. Female patients' and parents' assessment of deformity- and brace-related stress in the conservative treatment of adolescent idiopathic scoliosis. Spine 2012;37:1218–1223

17. Danielsson AJ, Romberg K, Nachemson AL. Spinal range of motion, muscle endurance, and back pain and function at least 20 years after fusion or brace treatment for adolescent idiopathic scoliosis: a case-control study. Spine 2006;31:275–283

18. Green DW, Lawhorne TW III, Widmann RF, et al. Long-term magnetic resonance imaging follow-up demonstrates minimal transitional level lumbar disc degeneration after posterior spine fusion for adolescent idiopathic scoliosis. Spine 2011;36:1948–1954

19. Kepler CK, Meredith DS, Green DW, Widmann RF. Long-term outcomes after posterior spine fusion for adolescent idiopathic scoliosis. Curr Opin Pediatr 2012;24:68–75

20. Mehlman CT, Araghi A, Roy DR. Hyphenated history: the Hueter-Volkmann law. Am J Orthop 1997;26:798–800

21. Nachlas IW, Borden JN. The cure of experimental scoliosis by directed growth control. J Bone Joint Surg Am 1951;33A:24–34

22. Smith AD, Von Lackum WH, Wylie R. An operation for stapling vertebral bodies in congenital scoliosis. J Bone Joint Surg Am 1954;36:342–348

23. Hershman SH, Park JJ, Lonner BS. Fusionless surgery for scoliosis. Bull Hosp Jt Dis (2013) 2013;71:49–53

24. Betz RR, Kim J, D'Andrea LP, Mulcahey MJ, Balsara RK, Clements DH. An innovative technique of vertebral body stapling for the treatment of patients with adolescent idiopathic scoliosis: a feasibility, safety, and utility study. Spine 2003;28:S255–S265

25. Betz RR, Ranade A, Samdani AF, et al. Vertebral body stapling: a fusionless treatment option for a growing child with moderate idiopathic scoliosis. Spine 2010;35:169–176

26. Uribe JS, Arredondo N, Dakwar E, Vale FL. Defining the safe working zones using the minimally invasive lateral retroperitoneal transpsoas approach: an anatomical study. J Neurosurg Spine 2010;13:260–266

27. Hunt KJ, Braun JT, Christensen BA. The effect of two clinically relevant fusionless scoliosis implant strategies on the health of the intervertebral disc: analysis in an immature goat model. Spine 2010;35:371–377

28. Betz RR, D'Andrea LP, Mulcahey MJ, Chafetz RS. Vertebral body stapling procedure for the treatment of scoliosis in the growing child. Clin Orthop Relat Res 2005;434:55–60

29. Cuddihy L, Danielsson AJ, Cahill PJ, et al. Vertebral body stapling versus bracing for patients with high-risk moderate idiopathic scoliosis. Biomed Res Int 2015;2015:438452

30. Lavelle WF, Samdani AF, Cahill PJ, Betz RR. Clinical outcomes of nitinol staples for preventing curve progression in idiopathic scoliosis. J Pediatr Orthop 2011;31(1, Suppl):S107–S113

31. Theologis AA, Cahill P, Auriemma M, Betz R, Diab M. Vertebral body stapling in children younger than 10 years with idiopathic scoliosis with curve magnitude of 30 degrees to 39 degrees. Spine 2013;38:E1583–E1588

32. Laituri CA, Schwend RM, Holcomb GW III. Thoracoscopic vertebral body stapling for treatment of scoliosis in young children. J Laparoendosc Adv Surg Tech A 2012;22:830–833

33. Trobisch PD, Samdani A, Cahill P, Betz RR. Vertebral body stapling as an alternative in the treatment of idiopathic scoliosis. Oper Orthop Traumatol 2011;23:227–231

34. Sanders JO, Khoury JG, Kishan S, et al. Predicting scoliosis progression from skeletal maturity: a simplified classification during adolescence. J Bone Joint Surg Am 2008;90:540–553

35. Newton PO, Farnsworth CL, Upasani VV, Chambers RC, Varley E, Tsutsui S. Effects of intraoperative tensioning of an anterolateral spinal tether on spinal growth modulation in a porcine model. Spine 2011;36:109–117

36. Braun JT, Ogilvie JW, Akyuz E, Brodke DS, Bachus KN. Creation of an experimental idiopathic-type scoliosis in an immature goat model using a flexible posterior asymmetric tether. Spine 2006;31:1410–1414

37. Braun JT, Akyuz E, Ogilvie JW, Bachus KN. The efficacy and integrity of shape memory alloy staples and bone anchors with ligament tethers in the fusionless treatment of experimental scoliosis. J Bone Joint Surg Am 2005;87:2038–2051

38. Newton PO, Upasani VV, Farnsworth CL, et al. Spinal growth modulation with use of a tether in an immature porcine model. J Bone Joint Surg Am 2008;90:2695–2706

39. Samdani AF, Ames RJ, Kimball JS, et al. Anterior vertebral body tethering for immature adolescent idiopathic scoliosis: one-year results on the first 32 patients. Eur Spine J 2015;24:1533–1539

40. Crawford CH III, Lenke LG. Growth modulation by means of anterior tethering resulting in progressive correction of juvenile idiopathic scoliosis: a case report. J Bone Joint Surg Am 2010;92:202–209

41. Newton PO, Yaszay B, Upasani VV, et al; Harms Study Group. Preservation of thoracic kyphosis is critical to maintain lumbar lordosis in the surgical treatment of adolescent idiopathic scoliosis. Spine 2010;35:1365–1370

42. Samdani AF, Ames RJ, Kimball JS, et al. Anterior vertebral body tethering for idiopathic scoliosis: two-year results. Spine 2014;39:1688–1693

43. Lonner BS, Lazar-Antman MA, Sponseller PD, et al. Multivariate analysis of factors associated with kyphosis maintenance in adolescent idiopathic scoliosis. Spine 2012;37:1297–1302

44. Sucato DJ, Agrawal S, O'Brien MF, Lowe TG, Richards SB, Lenke L. Restoration of thoracic kyphosis after operative treatment of adolescent idiopathic scoliosis: a multicenter comparison of three surgical approaches. Spine 2008;33:2630–2636

8

Long-Term Outcomes of Operative Management in Adolescent Idiopathic Scoliosis

Manabu Ito, Katsuhisa Yamada, and Ekkaphol Larpumnuayphol

▓ Introduction

The history of surgical treatment for adolescent idiopathic scoliosis (AIS) dates back 100 years ago.[1] After the advent of metallic spinal implants to correct spinal deformity in the middle of 20th century, the ability to correct spinal deformity has shown significant improvement.[2] Because most patients who undergo surgical treatment of AIS are younger than 20 years of age, their life expectancy after the primary surgery is longer than 50 years. To assess the lifelong value of deformity correction surgery for AIS, long-term follow-up studies on the effects of surgical treatment on patients' health-related parameters are indispensable. This chapter discusses the long-term clinical results of posterior and anterior surgery for AIS, based on studies with a minimum of 10 years of follow-up (**Table 8.1**). The parameters addressed include the correction rate of scoliotic deformity in each surgical procedure, surgery-related complications, rates and causes of revision surgery, long-term pulmonary function, and lumbar disk degeneration below the

lowest instrumented vertebra (LIV). The purpose of surgery in the adolescent is to prevent the consequences of deformity progression in adulthood. An important question remains regarding whether surgical treatment for AIS in children would prevent further progression of lumbar disk degeneration and residual spinal deformity and would help avoid severe deformity-related clinical problems in later years.

▓ History of Surgical Treatment for Adolescent Idiopathic Scoliosis

In the 1910s and 1920s, Russell Hibbs[1] performed long, uninstrumented in-situ posterior spinal fusion followed by a long-lasting immobilization with a cast. At the end of 1950s, Paul Harrington[2] was the first to use metallic spinal implants to correct spinal deformity and to enhance spinal fusion. He introduced a hook and rod system for concave-distraction

Table 8.1 Long-Term (> 10 Years) Follow-Up Reports of the Clinical Results of Posterior and Anterior Surgery for Adolescent Idiopathic Scoliosis

	PMID Number	Author	Journal	Year	Number of Subjects	Average Follow-Up Period in Years (Range)	Instrumentation
1	25996533	Iida T	Spine	2015	51 (Harrington 49, Luque 2)	22.6 (20–29)	Harrington or Luque
2	23595075	Sudo H	J Bone Joint Surg Am.	2013	32 (Lenke type 5C)	17.2 (12–23)	Anterior dual-rod instrumentation KASS
3	23169073	Sudo H	Spine	2013	25 (Lenke 1 MT)	15.2 (12–18)	Anterior spinal fusion (ASF) KASS
4	23064806	Min K	Eur Spine J	2013	48 Lenke 1 (A = 19, B = 8, C = 14), 7 Lenke 2 (lumbar modifier A = 2, B = 4, C = 1)	10	Posterior with all PS instrumentation
5	22037534	Akazawa T	Spine	2012	66	31.5 (21–41)	Posterior 58 (Harrington 45, Harrington with wiring 6, Chiba solid rod 7), anterior 8 (Dwyer 3, Zielke5)
6	21971127	Larson AN	Spine	2012	28 (AIS 1B,1C,3C) 19: selective thoracic fusion 9: long fusion	20 (14–24)	TSRH or CD instrumentation
7	21494198	Gitelman Y	Spine	2011	49	10.7 (8–16)	Group 1A (n = 17): open anterior spinal fusion/instrumentation; Group 1B (n = 9): combined open antero-posterior spinal fusion; Group 1C (n = 12): posterior spinal fusion/instrumentation with thoracoplasty; Group 2 (n = 11): posterior spinal fusion/instrumentation
8	21289549	Green DW	Spine	2011	20	11.8 (9.4–15.1)	Posterior fusion and segmental instrumentation (10: hybrid w/dual rods, PS, hook, wire; 9: dual rods all hook; 1: dual rods hook, wire)
9	20081516	Kelly DM	Spine	2010	18	16.97 (12–22)	Anterior spinal fusion (Dwyer, TSRH, or Zielke)
10	19910755	Bartie BJ	Spine	2009	171	19	Harrington
11	19752706	Takayama K	Spine	2009	32 (AIS 18)	21.1	Harrington: 7, CD: 8, Zielke: 2, Dwyer: 1
12	19713874	Takayama K	Spine	2009	32 (AIS 18)	21.1	Harrington: 7,CD: 8, Zielke: 2, Dwyer: 1
13	18519315	Helenius I	J Bone Joint Surg Am	2008	190	14.8	
14	17762812	Bjerkreim I	Spine	2007	44 single primary curves	10 (EQ, ODI), 5	CD

	PMID	Author	Journal	Year	N	Instrumentation	Follow-up (age)	Type
15	16924553	Benli IT	Eur Spine J	2007	109		11.3	TSRH
16	16449899	Danielsson AJ	Spine	2006	135		23.2 ± 1.6 (20.3–26.5)	Harrington
17	15864669	Mariconda M	Eur Spine J	2005	24		22.9 (20.2–27.3)	Single Harrington distraction rod
18	15706345	Helenius I	Spine	2005		Harrington:11 pairs, Cotrel-Dubousset:9 pairs, USS:10 pairs	Males 14.3 (6.7–23.0), Females 14.1 (6.4–23.7)	Harrington in 11 pairs, CD in 9 pairs, USS in 10 pairs
19	15526199	Niemeyer T	Int Orthop.	2005	41		23 (11–30)	Harrington
20	15371703	Remes V	Spine	2004		CD:57; USS:55	CD: 13.0 (11.2–15.0), USS 7.8 (6.1–10.5)	CD or USS
21	14668498	Helenius I	J Bone Joint Surg Am.	2003	57		13	CD
22	14501939	Danielsson AJ	Spine	2003	139		23.2 (20.3–26.6)	Harrington
23	12131746	Götze C	Spine	2002	82		16.7 (11–22)	Harrington
24	11805664	Helenius I	Spine	2002	78		20.8 (19.1–22.4)	Harrington
25	11563612	Danielsson AJ	Eur Spine J.	2001	146		23.3 (20.3–26.6)	Harrington
26	11389396	Padua R	Spine	2001	70		23.7 (15–28)	Harrington
27	11242379	Danielsson AJ	Spine	2001	139		23.2 (20.3–26.6)	Harrington
28	11259948	Danielsson AJ	Acta Radiol.	2001	32		23.2	Harrington
29	10984785	Pérez-Grueso FS	Spine	2000	35		Minimum 10	CD
30	7642667	Connolly PJ	J Bone Joint Surg Am	1995	83		12 (10–16)	Harrington
31	2326715	Kohler R	Spine	1990		21 lumbar/thoracolumbar	Minimum 10	Dwyer
32	2141336	Dickson JH	J Bone Joint Surg Am.	1990	206		21	Harrington

Abbreviations: AIS, adolescent idiopathic scoliosis; CD, Cotrel and Dubousset instrumentation; KASS, Kaneda Anterior Scoliosis System instrumentation; MT, midthoracic; ODI, Oswestry Disability Index; PS, pedicle screw; TSRH, Texas Scottish Rite Hospital instrumentation; USS, Universal Spine System instrumentation.

and convex-compression (**Fig. 8.1**). The next development was initiated by Eduardo Luque,[3] who uses sublaminar stainless-steel wires in combination with L-shaped rods in the 1970s. He used the implant for treatment of neuromuscular scoliosis and later for idiopathic scoliosis. The next generation of spinal instrumentation surgery was introduced by Cotrel and Dubousset[4] (CD instrumentation) at the beginning of the 1980s. They introduced a new concept of deformity correction, the rod rotation maneuver, to correct not only scoliosis but also rotational deformity of the deformed spine. CD instrumentation incorporates a frame construct consisting of two rods with multiple hooks (**Fig. 8.2**). Similar spinal instrumentation systems, including the Texas Scottish Rite Hospital (TSRH) instrumentation (Dallas, TX), Isola Spine System (Raynham, MA) (**Fig. 8.3**), and Moss-Miami system (DePuy, Warsaw, IN), had been introduced subsequently around the year 1990. These instruments consisted of two rods with multiple hooks, sublaminar wires, and pedicle screws. Modern sublaminar implants such as titanium cables and high-molecular polyester

bands have been developed recently to prevent metal corrosion and to protect the spinal cord.

After Suk et al[5] reported the use of pedicle screws (PSs) for scoliosis correction in 1995, PS instrumentation became a standard operative technique for idiopathic scoliosis around the year 2000 (**Fig. 8.4**). This transpedicular fixation systems enabled the surgeon to achieve better three-dimensional correction of scoliosis than with previous systems by allowing surgeons to use all available corrective techniques, such as derotation, translation, segmental distraction–compression, and in-situ bending of rods.[6] During the past 10 years, there have been significant developments in PS instrumentation with new correction techniques such as direct vertebral rotation (DVR),[7] simultaneous dual rod rotation, and others.[8]

With regard to anterior instrumentation for AIS, the Dwyer system was the first system introduced in 1970s.[9] Anterior systems consist of vertebral screws introduced on the convexity of the curve, with a flexible cable between the screws on which a compression force was applied on the convex side of the curve. This

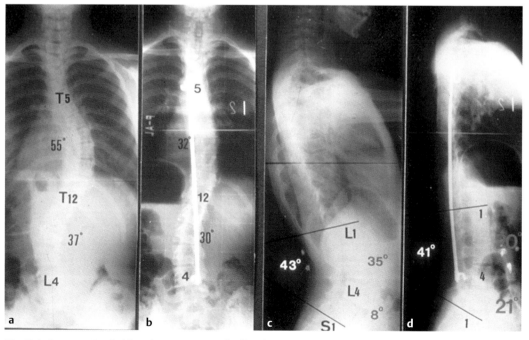

Fig. 8.1 Preoperative (**a,b**) and postoperative (**c,d**) radiographs of Harrington instrumentation (single distraction rod and two hooks).

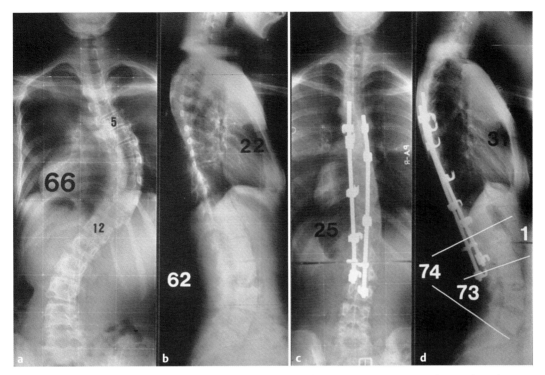

Fig. 8.2 Preoperative **(a,b)** and postoperative **(c,d)** radiographs of CD instrumentation (two rods and multiple hooks).

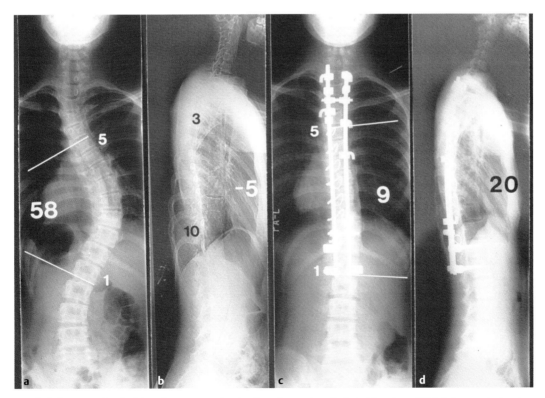

Fig. 8.3 Preoperative **(a,b)** and postoperative **(c,d)** radiographs of a hybrid system (ISOLA; two rods, hooks, sublaminar wires, and distal pedicle screws).

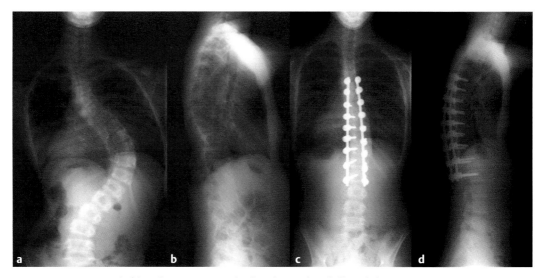

Fig. 8.4 Preoperative **(a,b)** and postoperative **(c,d)** radiographs of all–pedicle screw systems.

system was modified by Zielke with a threaded rod, and with a solid rod in the TSRH system. In the 1980s, the Kaneda device was developed for thoracolumbar-lumbar burst fractures. In 1989, the Kaneda device was modified to a multisegmental anterior spinal system and was used for correction of thoracolumbar scoliosis.[10] A unique character of Kaneda device was that it consisted of two rods and two vertebral screws in each vertebral body for biomechanical superiority and restoration of sagittal alignment of the spine (**Fig. 8.5**). As a minimally

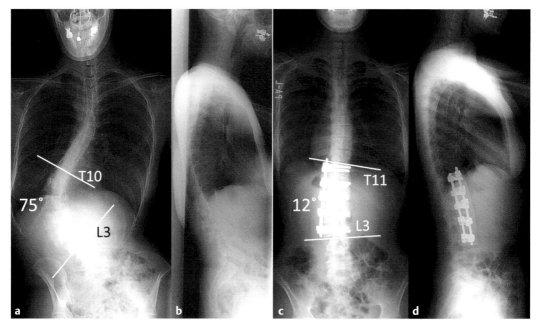

Fig. 8.5 Preoperative **(a,b)** and postoperative **(c,d)** radiographs of KASS (two vertebral screws and rods) for a thoracolumbar curve.

invasive surgery for thoracic curves, video-assisted thoracoscopic techniques (VATSs) have been utilized since the 1990s.[11] The technique involves anterior diskectomy and fusion with single rod instrumentation under endoscopic guidance, and it is commonly used for mild thoracic curves. Due to the recent development of posterior correction surgery, the current practice is that anterior surgery for AIS is conducted in selective cases with thoracolumbar and lumber curves.

Outcome of Posterior Procedures

Harrington Instrumentation

Lykissas et al[12] conducted a meta-analysis of 489 patients who underwent Harrington instrumentation (H-instrumentation) and were followed for an average of 20.7 years. The Cobb angle averaged 59.4 degrees (range, 55.8–63.0 degrees) before surgery and 41.8 degrees (range, 38.6–45.0 degrees) at the final follow-up. The average correction rate of the Cobb angle was 24.7%. Thoracic kyphosis averaged 35.3 degrees (range, 28.9–41.7 degrees) before surgery and 27.5 degrees (range, 20.6–34.7 degrees) at the final follow-up. The major correction force of H-instrumentation was distraction, so that there was a tendency of this system to create a flat back after surgery, which is a major limitation of H-instrumentation (**Fig. 8.1**). As for fusion with H-instrumentation, a 3.1% pseudarthrosis rate was reported by Lykiaas et al. Other studies reported fusion rates of H-instrumentation ranging from 93 to 100%. Mariconda et al[13] reported the functional outcome of H-instrumentation with the *Scoliosis Research Society* (SRS) score, which can be a maximum of 120 points. The SRS score in this study was 100.8 points, and there was no statistical difference between the patients and the controls in all domains. As for the rate of revision surgery, Lykissas et al reported that 38 of 459 patients (8.3%) had reoperations, some of which were for the following reasons: pseudar-

throsis in 10 patients, low back pain in seven, and rod removal for radicular pain in one. Danielsson et al[14] reported that eight patients (5.1%) required reoperations for hood dislodgment in three patients, flat back surgery in two, pseudarthrosis in one, and implant removal in two. Padua et al[15] reported that 48 of 70 patients (68.6%) required implant removal; the main reasons were implant-related pain in 10 patients, rod breakage in three, and progression of scoliosis in five.

CD Instrumentation

Lykissas et al[12] conducted a meta-analysis of mid- and long-term clinical results of 184 patients who underwent CD instrumentation (**Fig. 8.2**). The Cobb angle was 54.6 degrees (95% confidence interval, 52.9–56.2 degrees) before surgery and averaged 27.4 degrees (range, 21.9–33.0 degrees). The average correction rate of the Cobb angle was 49.8%. The preoperative thoracic kyphosis averaged 23.9 degrees (range, 14.4–33.4 degrees), and at final follow-up was 33.5 degrees (range, 30.8–36.2 degrees). Thoracic kyphosis was increased by 10 degrees after CD instrumentation. The successful fusion rate was 98.3%, and pseudarthrosis was observed in three of 177 patients (1.7%). Pérez-Grueso et al[16] reported that the functional outcomes of CD instrumentation with the SRS score were 96.7 ± 9.8 points, and there were no differences in all domains between the patients and the controls. Remes et al[17] reported that the average SRS score was 97 points, and six patients (11%) complained of frequent low-back pain. Regarding the long-term rate of reoperation, Bjerkreim et al[18] reported that one of 44 patients needed elongation of fusion levels due to postoperative trunk imbalance, and five needed their implants removed due to surgical-site infection (SSI). Remes et al reported that four of 57 patients underwent implant removal due to SSI, and one had postoperative neurologic deficits that were treated by changing the implant to H-instrumentation. Intraoperative lamina fracture was observed in four patients (7%), and dislodgment of caudal hook in six (10%).

Hybrid Instrumentation (Fig. 8.3)

Benli et al[19] reported the long-term clinical results in 109 patients treated with TSRH. The follow-up was 136.9 ± 12.7 months. The Cobb angle was 60.8 degrees before surgery and 28.2 degrees at the final follow-up. The average correction rate was 50.5% ± 23.1%. The average correction loss of the Cobb angle was 5.3 ± 5.8 degrees during follow-up. Another long-term follow-up study by Green et al[20] found that the Cobb angle before surgery was 55 ± 11 degrees, and at the final follow-up was 25 ± 10 degrees (correction rate of 55.5%). Their follow-up period was 11.8 years. The fusion rate was 90.8% in the Benli et al's study (nonunion in 10 of 109 patients) and 100% in the Green et al's study. As for the functional outcomes on the SRS-22 questionnaire, both studies found that the average score for each domain ranged from 3.6 to 4.6 points. There was a tendency for patients with a correction loss smaller than 10 degrees to show better scores on the domains of self-image and mental status than those whose correction loss was more than 10 degrees. As for reoperations, Benli et al reported that four patients (3.7%) had postoperative neurologic deficits treated with implant removal. Ten patients with nonunion underwent reoperation. Four patients had postoperative SSI (three early infection and one late infection) and underwent implant removal. In Green et al's study, no patient needed revision surgery. Three patients (2.8%) underwent scheduled implant removal due to the patients' demand.

All–Pedicle Screw System (Fig. 8.4)

Because the pedicle screw (PS) system does not have a long history, the reports of its long-term clinical results are limited. Min et al[21] reported that the correction rate in 48 patients with Lenke type 1 and 2 AIS curves was 55%. Their follow-up period was 10 years. Suk et al[6] reported the overall correction rate was 69% in 203 patients with King type 2, 3, 4, and 5 curves. There were several reports that the PS system had a tendency to decrease thoracic kyphosis. Min et al and Suk et al, however, reported that

the PS system did not decrease thoracic kyphosis but rather increased it by an average of 5 degrees. Both studies found that the fusion rate was 100%. And the functional clinical outcome (SRS-24 questionnaire, with a maximum score of 120 points) was 95 ± 22 points at 10 years postoperative. Min et al reported a reoperation rate of 12.5% (six patients) for implant removal due to SSI. Suk et al reported an SSI in 1.5% of patients in the early postoperative periods, and one patient required implant removal. In patients with SSI, however, solid fusion was obtained at the final follow-up. No patients needed reoperation due to junctional problems or neurologic complications in their series. Due to high correction rates of scoliosis for the all-PS system, however, postoperative shoulder imbalance has been reported in recent years. There are two solutions for this problem: (1) the upper instrumented vertebrae (UIVs) should include up to T2; and (2) decrease the correction rate for a major right convex thoracic curve so as not to elevate the left shoulder.

After rigid spinal fusion in patients with AIS, the incidence of junctional pathology in those treated with all-PS systems was reported to be comparable to that in those treated with hybrid systems that were biomechanically less rigid than the all-PS systems.[22] Another report found a correlation between preoperative proximal kyphosis above the UIV and its postoperative progression in AIS patients treated with spinal fusion.[23] The progression of junctional pathology following rigid spinal fusion may be a multifactorial event needing further research before conclusions can be drawn.

Anterior Procedures

Anterior procedures have been used for thoracolumbar curves and thoracic curves of AIS. Kohler et al[24] reported their long-term clinical results of Dwyer instrumentation for lumbar/ thoracolumbar curves. All patients were followed for more than 10 years. The Cobb angle was 56 degrees before surgery and 5 degrees after surgery (correction rate of 91.1%). During follow-up, a correction loss of more than 10 degrees was observed. Breakage of cables and nonunion were common in patients with significant correction loss exceeding 10 degrees. Kelly et al[25] reported their clinical results in 18 patients who underwent thoracolumbar fusion using Dwyer, TSRH, or Zielke instrumentation. The follow-up period averaged 17 years. The Cobb angle was 49.3 degrees before surgery and 25.6 degrees at the final follow-up (correction rate of 48%). Thoracic kyphosis was 21 degrees (range, 5–40 degrees) before surgery and 23 degrees (range, 13–37 degrees) at the final follow-up. Sudo et al[26] reported their long-term clinical results of 30 patients (Lenke type 5) who underwent thoracolumbar anterior surgery using a two-rod system (Kaneda Anterior Scoliosis System [KASS]) (**Fig. 8.5**). The average follow-up period was 17.2 years. The Cobb angle was 55.6 degrees before surgery and 11.3 degrees at the final follow-up (correction rate of 79.8%). The correction loss during follow-up was 3.4 degrees. Thoracic kyphosis (T5–12) was 12.8 degrees before surgery and 15.8 degrees at the final follow-up.

For thoracic curves, Tis et al[27] reported their clinical results of 85 patients (Lenke type 1) who underwent open anterior surgery using a single-rod system (open instrumented anterior spinal fusion [OASF]). The Cobb angle was 52 degrees before surgery and 25 degrees at the final follow-up (correction rate of 50%). Thoracic kyphosis was 28 ± 13 degrees initially and 38 ± 10 degrees at 5-year follow-up. Sudo et al[28] reported their clinical results of 25 patients (Lenke type 1) using a double-rod system (KASS). Their correction rate averaged 56.7% and their correction loss averaged 9.2 degrees. Thoracic kyphosis (T5–12) was 10.6 degrees before surgery and 20.5 degrees at the final follow-up. Their average follow-up period was 15.2 years.

A limited number of reports address the fusion rate after anterior surgery for AIS. Though Kohler et al[24] reported that one-level nonunion was common after Dwyer instrumentation, there was no precise description of the fusion rate in their report. Sudo et al[26] reported a fusion rate of 100% in Lenke type 5 and 96% (24/25 patients) in Lenke type 1.

To assess functional outcomes, Kelly et al[25] used the SRS-30 questionnaire, which has a maximum score of 115 points, and reported on average score of 98 points in their patients who were treated with anterior surgery. There was no precise information regarding the differences among implants. Sudo's paper showed an average score in each domain of all 30 domains of SRS30. The highest score is 5 and lowest is 1.[26,28]

Revision surgery was performed on two patients (11.1%) in the Kelly's series, in one patient for Dwyer screw breakage, and in the other for Zielke rod breakage. Three patients (4%) needed revision surgery in the Tis's series, including one for implant breakage and one for curve progression; although five patients experienced rod breakage and four had proximal screw pullout, additional surgery was not conducted on these patients. In the Sudo's series, two Lenke type 5 patients needed additional posterior surgery due to subjacent segment degeneration in one and progression of the thoracic curve in the other. Two Lenke type 1 patients required additional treatment; one patient needed posterior surgery due to nonunion, and the other needed implant removal due to an intermittent cough with hemoptysis caused by implant prominence into the thoracic cavity.

With regard to respiratory function tests, Sudo et al[26] reported that the average percent-predicted forced vital capacity (%FVC) and forced expiratory volume in 1 second (%FEV$_1$) were significantly decreased during a follow-up of more than 10 years (73% and 69%; $p = 0.0004$ and 0.0016, respectively) after open anterior surgery for the thoracic spine. No patient, however, had complaints related to the decreased pulmonary function. There was no adverse effect on pulmonary function after anterior open surgery for thoracolumbar/lumbar curves. Lonner et al[29] reported a contradictory result: open thoracotomy or thoracoplasty with resection of three to five ribs showed a significant decrease in pulmonary function 2 years after anterior surgery.[29]

Disk Degeneration in the Lumbar Spine

Nohara et al[30] investigated the incidence of lumbar disk degeneration (DD) in distal unfused segments and low back pain (LBP) in AIS patients. Their study included three groups: (1) surgery ($n = 52$), (2) nonsurgical mild scoliosis ($n = 45$), and (3) nonsurgical severe scoliosis ($n = 52$). All the patients were followed for more than 10 years. Radiographs and magnetic resonance imaging were used to evaluate the degree of DD in the lumbar spine. DD was observed in 61.5% in the surgery group, 47.7% in the nonsurgical mild scoliosis group, and 84.4% in the nonsurgical severe scoliosis group. LBP was observed in 51.9% in the surgical group, 64.4% in the nonsurgical mild scoliosis group, and 84.4% in the nonsurgical severe scoliosis group. No significant differences in DD and LBP were observed between the surgical group and the nonsurgical mild scoliosis group. There were significant differences, however, in DD and LBP between the surgical group and the nonsurgical severe scoliosis group. The results demonstrated that surgical treatment of AIS significantly decreased the incidence of DD and LBP after 10 years compared with the nonsurgical severe scoliosis group. The most frequent level of DD was the L5/S1 disk level in the surgery group, and L3/4 and L4/5 in the nonsurgical group. Green et al[20] reported the same result, that the most frequent level of DD (more than grade 3 in the Pfirrmann grading system) after surgical treatment was L5/S1, which was observed in 45% of their surgical treatment group (20 patients).

Respiratory Function

Gitelman et al[31] investigated long-term pulmonary function in two groups: group 1, patients with surgical procedures on the thoracic cavity; and group 2, patients with no surgical procedures on the thoracic cavity. They found that %FVC and %FEV_1 in group 1 showed a significant decrease at 10 years after surgery. In group 2, however, FVC showed a significant increase, and there was no change in %FVC and %FEV_1. They concluded that surgical procedures on the thoracic cavity would result in a long-term deterioration in pulmonary function. Saito et al[32] investigated the respiratory function of surgically treated AIS patients more than 10 years after surgery. Their study included

three groups: group 1, posterior corrective fusion ($n = 25$); group 2, posterior corrective fusion with thoracoplasty ($n = 10$); and group 3, combined open anteroposterior spinal fusion ($n = 13$). In groups 1 and 3, preoperative FVC and %FVC showed a significant increase at the final follow-up. One reason for this may be that posterior surgical correction of thoracic scoliosis was able to enlarge the thoracic cavity and ended up improving pulmonary function. In group 2, there was no difference in FVC and %FVC before surgery and at final follow-up. The authors concluded that surgical procedures on the chest wall such as thoracoplasty and anterior thoracotomy in posterior corrective surgery for AIS had no negative impact on pulmonary function at 10-year follow-up. Although there is some surgical invasiveness in the thoracic wall, correction of both severe spinal deformity and chest wall deformity has a long-term clinical benefit for pulmonary function of patients with severe thoracic deformity. Another study, however, reported that although open thoracotomy or thoracoplasty with resection of three to five ribs resulted in a significant decrease in pulmonary function at 2 years after anterior surgery with or without endoscopy, no significant decrease was observed in patients with thoracolumbar curves treated with a thoracolumbar approach.[29]

Revision Surgery

In 2006, Richards et al[33] reported the largest study (1,046 patients) of reoperations after primary spine fusion for AIS. They found a 12.9% reoperation rate over 15 years. A study by Luhmann et al[34] in 2009 reported a reoperation rate in spinal fusions in AIS of 3.9% (41/1,057 patients) at 5.7-year follow-up, which is more than three times lower than that found in the Richards study. Forty-seven additional procedures were performed within an average of 26 months after the primary surgery. Twenty of these procedures (43%) were revision spinal fusions for pseudarthrosis, uninstrumented curve progression, or junctional kyphosis; 16 (34%) were for SSI; seven (15%) were for implant removal due to pain and/or prominence; two (4%) were for revision of loosened implants;

and two (4%) were for elective thoracoplasties. The reoperation rates for different surgical procedures were 3.7% in posterior surgery, 4.3% in anterior surgery, and 4.1% in combined anterior-posterior surgery. There was no significant difference between surgical procedures. Multiple patient, surgeon, and institution factors are likely to account for differences in the reoperation rates after primary spinal fusion for AIS.

⦀ Chapter Summary

There is a 100-year history of surgical treatment for adolescent idiopathic scoliosis. Since the advent of metallic spinal implants to correct spinal deformity in the middle of the last century, the clinical results of surgical treatment for spinal deformity have shown a significant improvement. Average correction rates of each posterior spinal instrumentation surgery were 25% in Harrington instrumentation, 50% in CD instrumentation, 55% in Hybrid instrumentation, and 70% in the all-PS system. The correction rates of anterior surgery for AIS treated with KASS are 57% in thoracic curves and 80% in thoracolumbar/lumbar curves. Successful spinal fusion was achieved in 90 to 100% of patients treated either by posterior or anterior procedures. The reoperation rate after the primary scoliosis surgery ranged from 4 to 13%. The most frequent causes of reoperation were pseudarthrosis or curve progression in unfused segments in 43% of revision cases, followed by SSI in 34%, and implant-related pain in 15%. Comparing the incidence of lumbar DD and LBP between surgically treated patients and conservatively treated patients, the surgically treated group had significantly better functional outcomes during long-term follow-up. This is strong evidence that early corrective spinal surgery is of significant clinical benefit to AIS patients for the rest of their life. Surgical treatment for AIS, therefore, should be recommended to patients in a timely manner when their curves have progressed and reached surgical indications. Although anterior open surgery for thoracic curves had some negative long-term effects on pulmonary function, patients did not have complaints regarding their activities of daily living. For severe thoracic curves, anterior release through thoracotomy combined with posterior instrumentation surgery was able to increase the thoracic volume, which finally overcame the disadvantages of surgical invasion of the thoracic wall.

Pearls

- All-PS instrumentation has achieved a high correction rate (70%) of scoliotic deformity.
- Restoration of physiological thoracic kyphosis has become possible because of recent advances in posterior correction surgery using PSs.
- Anterior corrective surgery is an excellent option for flexible thoracolumbar/lumbar curves.
- Appropriate surgical treatment for AIS prevents further progression of lumbar disk degeneration below the LIV, as compared with nonoperative care, and decreases the risk of low back pain in later years. Fusion to L5 may be the exception to this finding.
- The fusion rate of recent all-PS systems is close to 100%, and the long-term reoperation rate is less than 13%.

Pitfalls

- Distraction devices such as Harrington instrumentation decreases thoracic kyphosis and tends to produce a flat back.
- All pedicle screw instrumentation has a tendency to create a shoulder imbalance after surgery due to its high correction rate.
- Although open anterior surgery for the thoracic spine may decrease long-term pulmonary function, patients do not have complaints regarding their activities of daily living.
- Common reasons for reoperation after surgical treatment for AIS are pseudarthrosis and progression below the LIV, followed by surgical-site infection and pain related to spinal implants.

References
Five Must-Read References

1. Hibbs RA. An operation for progressive spinal deformities. NY Med 1911;93:1013
2. Harrington PR. Treatment of scoliosis. Correction and internal fixation by spine instrumentation. J Bone Joint Surg Am 1962;44-A:591–610
3. Luque ER. Segmental spinal instrumentation for correction of scoliosis. Clin Orthop Relat Res 1982;163: 192–198
4. Cotrel Y, Dubousset J, Guillaumat M. New universal instrumentation in spinal surgery. Clin Orthop Relat Res 1988;227:10–23
5. Suk SI, Lee CK, Kim WJ, Chung YJ, Park YB. Segmental pedicle screw fixation in the treatment of thoracic idiopathic scoliosis. Spine 1995;20:1399–1405
6. Suk SI, Lee SM, Chung ER, Kim JH, Kim SS. Selective thoracic fusion with segmental pedicle screw fixation in the treatment of thoracic idiopathic scoliosis: more than 5-year follow-up. Spine 2005;30:1602–1609
7. Lee SM, Suk SI, Chung ER. Direct vertebral rotation: a new technique of three-dimensional deformity correction with segmental pedicle screw fixation in adolescent idiopathic scoliosis. Spine 2004;29:343–349
8. Ito M, Abumi K, Kotani Y, et al. Simultaneous double rod rotation technique in posterior instrumentation surgery for correction of adolescent idiopathic scoliosis. Technical note. JNS:Spine 2010;12:293–300
9. Dwyer AF, Newton NC, Sherwood AA. An anterior approach to scoliosis. A preliminary report. Clin Orthop Relat Res 1969;62:192–202
10. Kaneda K, Shono Y, Satoh S, Abumi K. New anterior instrumentation for the management of thoracolumbar and lumbar scoliosis. Application of the Kaneda two-rod system. Spine 1996;21:1250–1261, discussion 1261–1262
11. Lenke LG. Anterior endoscopic discectomy and fusion for adolescent idiopathic scoliosis. Spine 2003;28(15 Suppl):S36–S43
12. Lykissas MG, Jain VV, Nathan ST, et al. Mid- to long-term outcomes in adolescent idiopathic scoliosis after instrumented posterior spinal fusion: a meta-analysis. Spine 2013;38:E113–E119
13. Mariconda M, Galasso O, Barca P, Milano C. Minimum 20-year follow-up results of Harrington rod fusion for idiopathic scoliosis. Eur Spine J 2005;14:854–861
14. Danielsson AJ, Romberg K, Nachemson AL. Spinal range of motion, muscle endurance, and back pain and function at least 20 years after fusion or brace treatment for adolescent idiopathic scoliosis: a case-control study. Spine 2006;31:275–283
15. Padua R, Padua S, Aulisa L, et al. Patient outcomes after Harrington instrumentation for idiopathic scoliosis: a 15- to 28-year evaluation. Spine 2001;26:1268–1273
16. Pérez-Grueso FS, Fernández-Baíllo N, Arauz de Robles S, García Fernández A. The low lumbar spine below Cotrel-Dubousset instrumentation: long-term findings. Spine 2000;25:2333–2341
17. Remes V, Helenius I, Schlenzka D, Yrjönen T, Ylikoski M, Poussa M. Cotrel-Dubousset (CD) or Universal Spine System (USS) instrumentation in adolescent idiopathic scoliosis (AIS): comparison of midterm clinical, functional, and radiologic outcomes. Spine 2004;29:2024–2030
18. Bjerkreim I, Steen H, Brox JI. Idiopathic scoliosis treated with Cotrel-Dubousset instrumentation: evaluation 10 years after surgery. Spine 2007;32:2103–2110
19. Benli IT, Ates B, Akalin S, Citak M, Kaya A, Alanay A. Minimum 10 years follow-up surgical results of adolescent idiopathic scoliosis patients treated with TSRH instrumentation. Eur Spine J 2007;16:381–391
20. Green DW, Lawhorne TW III, Widmann RF, et al. Long-term magnetic resonance imaging follow-up demonstrates minimal transitional level lumbar disc degeneration after posterior spine fusion for adolescent idiopathic scoliosis. Spine 2011;36:1948–1954
21. Min K, Sdzuy C, Farshad M. Posterior correction of thoracic adolescent idiopathic scoliosis with pedicle screw instrumentation: results of 48 patients with minimal 10-year follow-up. Eur Spine J 2013;22:345–354
22. Kim YJ, Lenke LG, Kim J, et al. Comparative analysis of pedicle screw versus hybrid instrumentation in posterior spinal fusion of adolescent idiopathic scoliosis. Spine 2006;31:291–298
23. Lee GA, Betz RR, Clements DH III, Huss GK. Proximal kyphosis after posterior spinal fusion in patients with idiopathic scoliosis. Spine 1999;24:795–799
24. Kohler R, Galland O, Mechin H, Michel CR, Onimus M. The Dwyer procedure in the treatment of idiopathic scoliosis. A 10-year follow-up review of 21 patients. Spine 1990;15:75–80
25. Kelly DM, McCarthy RE, McCullough FL, Kelly HR. Long-term outcomes of anterior spinal fusion with instrumentation for thoracolumbar and lumbar curves in adolescent idiopathic scoliosis. Spine 2010; 35:194–198
26. Sudo H, Ito M, Kaneda K, Shono Y, Abumi K. Long-term outcomes of anterior dual-rod instrumentation for thoracolumbar and lumbar curves in adolescent idiopathic scoliosis: a twelve to twenty-three-year follow-up study. J Bone Joint Surg Am 2013;95:e49
27. Tis JE, O'Brien MF, Newton PO, et al. Adolescent idiopathic scoliosis treated with open instrumented

anterior spinal fusion: five-year follow-up. Spine 2010;35:64–70

28. Sudo H, Ito M, Kaneda K, Shono Y, Takahata M, Abumi K. Long-term outcomes of anterior spinal fusion for treating thoracic adolescent idiopathic scoliosis curves: average 15-year follow-up analysis. Spine 2013;38:819–826

29. Lonner BS, Auerbach JD, Estreicher MB, et al. Pulmonary function changes after various anterior approaches in the treatment of adolescent idiopathic scoliosis. J Spinal Disord Tech 2009;22:551–558

30. Nohara A, Kawakami N, Tsuji T, et al. Intervertebral disc degeneration during postoperative follow-up more than 10 years after corrective surgery in idiopathic scoliosis: comparison between patients with and without surgery. J Spine Res 2013;4:1651–1655 (Japanese)

31. Gitelman Y, Lenke LG, Bridwell KH, Auerbach JD, Sides BA. Pulmonary function in adolescent idiopathic scoliosis relative to the surgical procedure: a 10-year follow-up analysis. Spine 2011;36:1665–1672

32. Saito T, Tsuji T, Suzuki O, et al. Pulmonary function in idiopathic scoliosis relative to the surgical procedure: Long time follow-up analysis. J. Spine Res 2014;5:1528–1532 (Japanese)

33. Richards BS, Hasley BP, Casey VF. Repeat surgical interventions following "definitive" instrumentation and fusion for idiopathic scoliosis. Spine 2006;31:3018–3026

34. Luhmann SJ, Lenke LG, Bridwell KH, Schootman M. Revision surgery after primary spine fusion for idiopathic scoliosis. Spine 2009;34:2191–2197

9

Revision Pediatric Spinal Deformity Surgery

Lawrence G. Lenke

Introduction

The need for revision surgery is an important complication in pediatric spinal deformity surgery, and a significant consideration in the cost and risk of surgery in the adolescent. The need for revision surgery in the pediatric spinal deformity patient is certainly much less common than in the adult deformity population. However, there are a variety of circumstances that require revision surgery (or multiple revision surgeries) in this patient group. The diagnoses requiring revision surgery can be divided into early and late etiologies. Suboptimal correction, wound issues, implant issues, and neural issues typically occur and need treatment in the early postoperative period. Later, issues such as deformity progression in the unfused spine, pseudarthrosis, and junctional pathology can occur. However, wound and implant issues have shown up many years after surgery, and junctional problems have been seen early in some patients. The key is encouraging regular follow-up visits after surgery and carefully evaluating the patient clinically and radiographically. This chapter discusses revision surgery in the pediatric patient with spinal deformity, with a focus on both prevention of occurrence and surgical strategies for revision.

Suboptimal Clinical or Radiographic Outcome

The selection of specific operative treatments for pediatric patients with various spinal deformities is quite variable. Certainly, in the current era of segmental pedicle screw fixation, rigid posterior-only constructs with attendant thorough spinal fusion are the mainstay of treatment that can be applied to any pediatric spinal deformity. However, often these are combined with various posterior-based spinal osteotomies for increased deformity correction. Alternatively, anterior release of the spine, which is now less common, is still performed by some surgeons for severe coronal or sagittal plane deformities, and to limit fusion levels in some type 1 and 5 Lenke curves. The challenges of managing a deformity patient increase as the size and stiffness of the operative curve(s) increase, leading to a higher rate of complications and the potential need for revision surgery.

In the adolescent idiopathic scoliosis (AIS) population, the need for revision surgery up to 20 years later varies considerably, ranging from ~ 13% in one series to just under 4% in another series from busy pediatric deformity centers.[1,2] The reasons for revision surgery were quite similar, with the most prevalent being problems with instrumentation constructs or fusion, leading to revisions for implant dislodgement, curve progression, truncal imbalance, and pseudarthrosis. However, these series were accrued prior to the common usage of segmental pedicle screw constructs, which have a far lower revision rate than do hook or hybrid constructs in the pediatric deformity surgical population.[3] The most important component to any deformity construct is secure and solid fixation at the most cephalad and caudad ends of the construct. We recommend at least four solid screw anchors at the ends of the construct, and six if the patient or deformity requirements are more substantial. The quality of fixation is as important as the quantity, if not more so. Thus, secure screw purchase must be confirmed intraoperatively following both implant and construct placement. This should be performed by both radiographic and physical means (i.e., in vivo construct security assessment) on every surgical procedure. If a construct is not secure on the operating room table, it will certainly not be secure when the patient is upright and ambulating.

The classification of deformity and the choice of fusion levels are important considerations in limiting the risk of revision surgery. Classifying and then appropriately treating AIS patients remains controversial. Although the Lenke AIS classification system[4] is the most widely used, there are known "rule breakers" where the recommended fusion regions may vary from inclusion of the structural curves alone. The most problematic areas are optimizing clinical shoulder balance in main thoracic type 1 and double thoracic type 2 curves.[5] There are patients with clinically level shoulders, a large main thoracic curve, and a nonstructural proximal thoracic curve (i.e., a type 1 main thoracic curve) in which the left shoulder will be elevated postoperatively due to the marked correction of the main thoracic curve when the upper instrumented vertebra (UIV) is T4 or T5. This can also become problematic when the UIV is T2 or T3 if the shoulders are not well aligned during the operative proce-

dure. The production of a "high left shoulder" in AIS surgery is probably the most common suboptimal condition postoperatively, but only a fraction of those patients will require revision surgery for this malalignment.

Another quite controversial area is the decision to perform a selective thoracic fusion (STF) for Lenke 1C, 2C or even 3C and 4C curves. Although it is often advisable to try to leave the nonstructural lumbar curve unfused for functional reasons, postoperative decompensation can occur in the unfused lumbar spine requiring revision surgery.[6] The two most common reasons are inappropriate selection of patients to undergo an STF and overcorrecting the thoracic curve beyond which the unfused lumbar curve can accommodate.[7] In addition, patients with inadequate, or excessive, sagittal plane restoration of the thoracic or thoracolumbar region and those with subtle connective tissue laxity are also prone to postoperative problems including junctional kyphosis.[8] Patients with selective thoracic fusion and postoperative coronal or sagittal plane decompensation that does not spontaneously correct over time may require revision surgery that extends the thoracic instrumentation and fusion to the low lumbar region, either L3 or more commonly L4.

The surgical treatment of skeletally immature patients, whether for AIS or for other diagnoses, is challenging, and may require revision surgery if subsequent growth leads to progressive deformity. The risks of adding on to the upper or lower end of the construct, or progression of the apical segments leading to a crankshaft phenomenon, or both, are important causes of revision surgery in patients with significant spinal growth remaining.[9] Revision surgery usually requires extension of the lowest instrumented vertebra (LIV) to L4 or even L5 in some circumstances. Interestingly, at my center we have not seen many problems with lumbar curve progression following successful STF in the immature patient; conversely, we have seen problems with selective lumbar fusions in which thoracic curve progression in the immature patient that is recalcitrant to postoperative bracing attempts require fusion and instrumentation of the thoracic curve. Revision requires the extension of the lumbar construct to the upper thoracic region, with segmental apical screw fixation used to minimize progressive thoracic deformity with continued growth. This is illustrated in **Fig. 9.1** in a skeletally immature girl who had a 55-degree Lenke 5CN AIS deformity. After undergoing a posterior selective lumbar instrumentation and fusion from T11 to L4, she had progression of her thoracic curve from 50 degrees at 2 months postoperative to 65 degrees at 2 years. Her

lumbar curve increased from 39 to 49 degrees and she had increased her thoracic kyphosis to +69 degrees as well. She underwent a revision posterior procedure consisting of implant removal and fusion exploration (she was solidly fused from T11 to L4), then multiple posterior column osteotomies (PCOs) of the apex of both the thoracic and lumbar curves, with definitive instrumentation and fusion from T3 to L5. As a general rule to follow, fusing the immature spine short will always run the risk of unfused curve progression, and patients and parents need to understand this ahead of time to avoid any surprises postoperatively.[9]

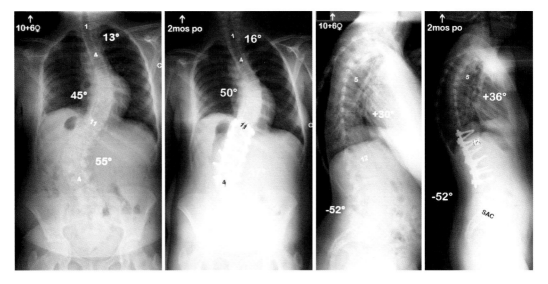

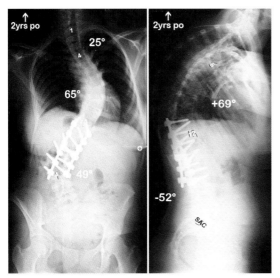

Fig. 9.1 This 10 year + 6 month female had a 55-degree Lenke 5CN adolescent idiopathic scoliosis (AIS) deformity. She underwent a posterior selective lumbar instrumentation and fusion from T11 to L4 (she has six functioning lumbar vertebrae). **(a)** At 2 months postoperative, her lumbar curve was stable at 39 degrees, but her thoracic curve had started to increase to 50 degrees. **(b)** By 2 years postoperative with continued growth, her thoracic curve had increased to 65 degrees, her lumbar curve to 49 degrees, and she had increased her thoracic kyphosis to +69 degrees.

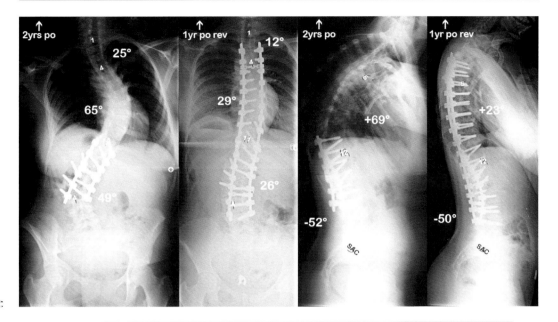

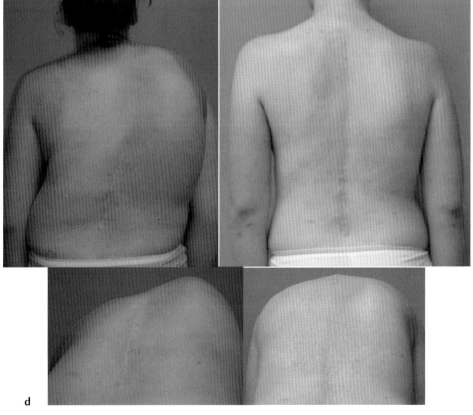

d

Fig. 9.1 (*continued*) **(c)** She thus underwent a revision posterior procedure consisting of implant removal and fusion exploration (she was solidly fused from T11 to L4), then multiple posterior column osteotomies (PCOs) of the apex of both the thoracic and lumbar curves, and definitive instrumentation and fusion from T3 to L5. Her postoperative radiographic alignment is excellent. **(d)** Her pre- and post-revision clinical photos demonstrate her clinical correction.

Wound-Related Issues

The occurrence of acute and chronic deep wound infections is still a common source of revision surgery in the pediatric deformity population. The incidence is much higher in the neuromuscular population than seen in AIS surgery, but no patient is completely risk free. The standardization of appropriately timed intravenous antibiotics used perioperatively along with the common application of intra-site vancomycin powder has certainly lowered the acute deep wound infection rates in many centers around the world. However, the occurrence of chronic, often indolent infections from normal skin flora such as *Propionibacterium acnes* continues to be a rare but troubling complication that usually necessitates complete implant removal for eradication.[10] Early and aggressive irrigation and debridement of suspicious wounds with postoperative suction wound drainage with implant preservation is the mainstay of treatment with long-term intravenous and then oral antibiotics prescribed based on cultures and sensitivities. In the neuromuscular population, the use of prophylactic gram-negative perioperative antibiotic coverage along with the application of skin glue to the wound edges to prevent secondary urinary or fecal local contamination has helped lessen the acute infection rate. In the most complex patients such as those with high-level myelomeningocele and poor tissue coverage, utilizing the skills of plastic surgeons for complex wound closures has aided in successful wound healing in these challenging patients.

Implant-Related Issues With or Without Pseudarthrosis

Revision surgery is often needed for issues related to instrumentation. The spectrum of problems range from implant prominence to dislodgment to breakage with or without pseudarthrosis. Implant prominence nearly always occurs at the convex apex of the thoracic region in thin patients with an under-corrected apical deformity. The use of monoaxial or lower profile implants can help minimize this problem. Implant prominence due to proximal or distal implant pullout or dislodgment is a common reason for revision surgery at the upper and lower instrumented segments. This problem is much more common with kyphotic or kyphoscoliotic conditions, especially with constructs that are too short above or below, or with suboptimal purchase of the cephalad/caudad anchors following aggressive deformity correction.[2] Revision surgery in these cases can be challenging, as the old implant anchors have often destroyed or eroded the pertinent bony anatomy, rendering revision at those levels difficult if not impossible, so extension for several levels above and below is often required. In addition, the primary deformity often needs to be addressed with correction techniques using spinal osteotomies, including vertebral column resection (VCR) surgery, to avoid similar implant issues in the future. Often, preoperative halo-gravity traction (HGTx) may be helpful to reduce proximal thoracic or cervicothoracic kyphotic deformities prior to the revision surgery. This was the case in a 15-year-old girl with neurofibromatosis (**Fig. 9.2**). She had a long history of thoracic kyphoscoliosis treated with two prior anterior spinal fusions and five prior posterior instrumentation/fusions, starting with in situ fusion as a young child, with ultimate posterior implant removal for prominence and progressive deformity. She eventually developed 110 degrees of scoliosis and 160 degrees of kyphosis. Her three-dimensional computed tomography (CT) scan and magnetic resonance imaging (MRI) demonstrated the severely distorted nature of her deformity, with tenting of her spinal cord at the apex of her kyphosis. She underwent several weeks of HGTx followed by a three-level VCR with posterior instrumentation and fusion from C7 to L3.

Neural Complications

The goal of spinal deformity corrective surgery is to avoid any neural complications

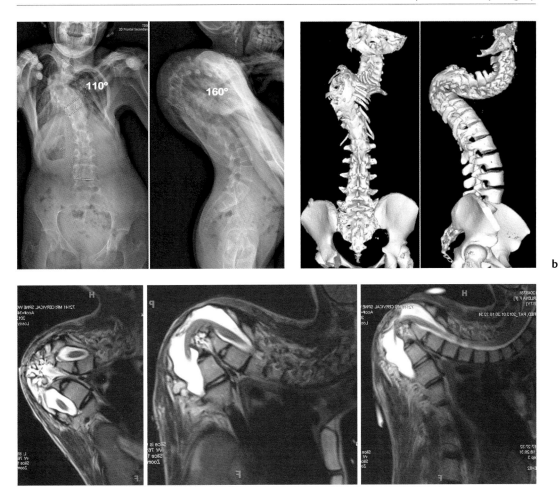

b

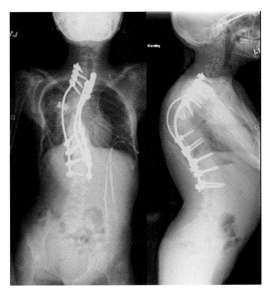

Fig. 9.2 A 15-year-old girl with neurofibromatosis had a long history of thoracic kyphoscoliosis treated with two prior anterior spinal fusions and five prior posterior instrumentation/fusions, starting with in situ fusion as a young child, with ultimate posterior implant removal for prominence. **(a)** Subsequently, her deformity progressed to 110 degrees of scoliosis and 160 degrees of kyphosis. **(b)** A 3D CT scan depicts the severely distorted nature of her deformity and prior posterior fusion attempts. **(c)** A preoperative sagittal thoracic MRI demonstrates the severe kyphotic angulation that is tenting her spinal cord at the apex where the cord is draped over the three apical vertebral bodies, T5, T6, and T7. **(d)** She underwent a three-level vertebral column resection (VCR) and posterior instrumentation and fusion from C7 to L3. Postoperative X-rays show markedly improved coronal and sagittal plane alignment and correction. (*continued on page 82*)

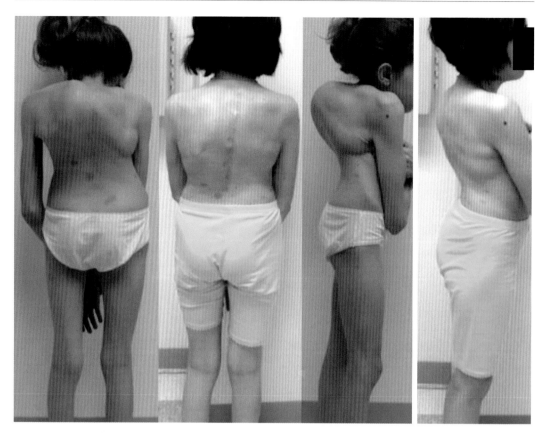

e

Fig. 9.2 (*continued*) **(e)** Pre- and postoperative photos demonstrate the dramatic correction of her truncal deformity.

postoperatively with the universal use of intraoperative monitoring (IOM) techniques of the spinal cord and nerve roots.[11] The intraoperative real-time warning of actual or impending neural complications can often be reversed by a thorough and thoughtful approach to improving the data, meeting warning criteria or actually being completely lost.[12] The goal is to reverse the data degradation to get as close to the baseline tracings as possible, as this has the best chance of returning patients to their baseline neural function postoperatively. However, although current IOM techniques are excellent at predicting spinal cord deficits, they are not as sensitive or specific for peripheral nerve issues, the most common one being postoperative radiculopathy from malpositioned pedicle screws.[13] Revision surgery for removal or redirection of a medially directed pedicle screw is probably the most common neural reason for returning the patient to the operating room. In addition, pedicle screws that are long with close proximity to the great vessels or other viscera, may require postoperative adjustment or removal. Very rarely, a pediatric patient may develop a postoperative delayed spinal cord deficit that demands immediate attention and return to the operating room for treatment that often entails spinal cord decompression of postoperative impingement from a hematoma, from other substances such as gelatin matrix material, from residual bone/disk fragments following osteotomy surgery, or for correction of junctional pathology. The decision to perform postoperative imaging such as CT or MRI scans is an individual one based on many factors, but with an evolving spinal cord deficit, returning to the operating room should be prompt and is usually beneficial once the cause of the delayed neural deficit is determined.

Junctional Pathology

The cephalad and caudad aspects of constructs are prone to postoperative problems, especially with correction of kyphotic spinal deformities. The problem of junctional kyphosis has been intensified by the use of powerful pedicle screws and osteotomy procedures that allow kyphosis correction often beyond what is physiological for the patient.[14] The most common junctional problem seen is proximal junctional kyphosis (PJK), which is defined as an increase of 10 degrees or more in the Cobb measurement from the UIV to the upper end plate of the UIV plus two vertebrae.[15] Most cases of PJK in the pediatric postoperative population are radiographic anomalies that have little clinical significance. However, more severe PJK deformities of more that 20 or 30 degrees in the Cobb measurement often produce clinical symptoms of pain and deformity in the cephalad region of the construct.[16] Proximal junctional kyphosis may involve mechanisms such as loss of fixation of the initial construct, fracture at or above the UIV, or subluxations of the supra-adjacent vertebra above the UIV. In rare circumstances, myelopathy from angular tenting of the spinal cord across a severe PJK may develop.

The treatment of PJK causing enough clinical symptoms or radiographic deformity to warrant revision surgery entails determining the proper revision UIV and correcting any associated kyphotic deformity. The deformity correction can be aided by preliminary HGTx, which is especially beneficial with more cephalad PJK issues involving the cervical or cervicothoracic region, but can also help proximal thoracic PJK deformities as well. A useful guide to selecting the revision UIV is to instrument/fuse across the first lordotic disk going cephalad, similar to what is done when choosing an LIV for kyphotic realignments.[17] At a minimum, including all kyphotic disks in the revision PJK construct is mandatory, and getting close to the first lordotic disk is recommended to avoid a recurrent PJK. We prefer secure pedicle screw implants in both primary kyphotic deformities and revision kyphotic deformities treated for PJK.[16]

Distal junctional problems in scoliosis or kyphosis surgery are usually related to choosing an LIV level that is too cephalad or to having insufficient caudal fixation.[18] Certainly the use of pedicle screws has lessened the occurrence as compared with hook or wire fixation techniques as caudal anchors.[3] However, caudal pedicle screw constructs need to be well positioned with a firm three-column purchase of the LIV to support the often significant load at the bottom of deformity constructs. Revision usually entails extending the construct distal at least one more level and occasionally supplementing with infralaminar hooks or even an interbody fusion of the lowest fused level if required.

Chapter Summary

Revision pediatric spinal deformity surgery is required for a variety of indications. It is important to determine the underlying prior pathology and prior treatment(s), and to develop a rational plan for the revision surgery that provides the best chance of fixing the presenting pathology at revision and of avoiding further problems and future surgeries. Although less commonly needed than adult spinal deformity revision surgery, revision surgery in the pediatric patient is an important and significant clinical problem, and these pediatric patients deserve our best efforts to safely perform their revision procedures while optimizing their outcomes.

Surgeons need to be mindful of potential adverse occurrences that may lead to revision surgery when planning pediatric spine surgery. One needs to have a clear surgical plan regarding the type and levels for the fusion and instrumentation, leaving the adolescent with an adequately supported and balanced spine. This chapter discussed the postoperative problems that can develop in the pediatric population, requiring further surgical intervention, with a focus on both prevention of occurrence and treatment of the established problem.

Pearls

◆ It is important to thoroughly assess each pediatric spinal deformity patient with appropriate radiographs and other imaging to understand the pathoanatomy.

◆ Classifying AIS by the Lenke system provides guidance on the regions of the spine to be fused and also provides a complete two-dimensional radiographic analysis.

◆ It is essential to ascertain why a revision surgery is needed by reviewing prior images and developing a strategy to avoid further problems.

Pitfalls

◆ One must be very careful with skeletally immature patients who can progress their deformity postoperatively with continued spinal growth.

◆ Junctional deformities developing either proximal or distal to the instrumentation and fusion following marked sagittal plane correction can lead to revision surgeries, especially if there is inadequate fixation.

◆ Removing spinal instrumentation, even in the face of a "solid fusion," can lead to progressive deformity by bending or breaking of the actual fusion mass and should be avoided.

References

Five Must-Read References

1. Richards BS, Hasley BP, Casey VF. Repeat surgical interventions following "definitive" instrumentation and fusion for idiopathic scoliosis. Spine 2006;31:3018–3026

2. Luhmann SJ, Lenke LG, Bridwell KH, Schootman M. Revision surgery after primary spine fusion for idiopathic scoliosis. Spine 2009;34:2191–2197

3. Kuklo TR, Potter BK, Lenke LG, Polly DW Jr, Sides B, Bridwell KH. Surgical revision rates of hooks versus hybrid versus screws versus combined anteroposterior spinal fusion for adolescent idiopathic scoliosis. Spine 2007;32:2258–2264

4. Lenke LG, Betz RR, Harms J, et al. Adolescent idiopathic scoliosis: a new classification to determine extent of spinal arthrodesis. J Bone Joint Surg Am 2001;83-A:1169–1181

5. Luhmann SJ, Lenke LG, Erickson M, Bridwell KH, Richards BS. Correction of moderate (<70 degrees) Lenke 1A and 2A curve patterns: comparison of hybrid and all-pedicle screw systems at 2-year follow-up. J Pediatr Orthop 2012;32:253–258

6. Skaggs DL, Seehausen DA, Yamaguchi KT Jr, et al. Assessment of the lowest instrumented vertebra tilt on radiographic measurements in Lenke "C" modifier curves undergoing selective thoracic fusion in adolescent idiopathic scoliosis. Spine Deform 2016;4:125–130

7. Crawford CH III, Lenke LG, Sucato DJ, et al. Selective thoracic fusion in Lenke 1C curves: prevalence and criteria. Spine 2013;38:1380–1385

8. Gomez JA, Matsumoto H, Colacchio ND, et al. Risk factors for coronal decompensation after posterior spinal instrumentation and fusion for adolescent idiopathic scoliosis. Spine Deform 2014;2:380–385

9. Chang MS, Bridwell KH, Lenke LG, et al. Predicting the outcome of selective thoracic fusion in false double major lumbar "C" cases with 5- to 24-year follow-up. Spine 2010;35:2128–2133

10. Hedequist D, Haugen A, Hresko T, Emans J. Failure of attempted implant retention in spinal deformity delayed surgical site infections. Spine 2009;34:60–64

11. Thuet ED, Winscher JC, Padberg AM, et al. Validity and reliability of intraoperative monitoring in pediatric spinal deformity surgery: a 23-year experience of 3436 surgical cases. Spine 2010;35:1880–1886

12. Vitale MG, Skaggs DL, Pace GI, et al. Best practices in intraoperative neuromonitoring in spine deformity surgery: Development of an intraoperative checklist to optimize response. Spine Deform 2014;2:333–339

13. Raynor BL, Padberg AM, Lenke LG, et al. Failure of intraoperative monitoring to detect postoperative neurologic deficits: A 25-year experience in 12,375 spinal surgeries. Spine 2016;41:1387–1393; [Epub ahead of print]

14. Kim HJ, Bridwell KH, Lenke LG, et al. Patients with proximal junctional kyphosis requiring revision surgery have higher postoperative lumbar lordosis and larger sagittal balance corrections. Spine 2014;39:E576–E580

15. Cho SK, Kim YJ, Lenke LG. Proximal junctional kyphosis following spinal deformity surgery in the pediatric patient. J Am Acad Orthop Surg 2015;23:408–414

16. Kim YJ, Lenke LG, Bridwell KH, et al. Proximal junctional kyphosis in adolescent idiopathic scoliosis after 3 different types of posterior segmental spinal

instrumentation and fusions: incidence and risk factor analysis of 410 cases. Spine 2007;32:2731–2738

17. Kim YJ, Bridwell KH, Lenke LG, Kim J, Cho SK. Proximal junctional kyphosis in adolescent idiopathic scoliosis following segmental posterior spinal instrumentation and fusion: minimum 5-year follow-up. Spine 2005;30:2045–2050

18. Lowe TG, Lenke L, Betz R, et al. Distal junctional kyphosis of adolescent idiopathic thoracic curves following anterior or posterior instrumented fusion: incidence, risk factors, and prevention. Spine 2006; 31:299–302

10

Spondylolisthesis: Classification and Natural History

Kariman Abelin-Genevois and Pierre Roussouly

Introduction

L5-S1 spondylolisthesis is the forward displacement or slippage of the fifth lumbar vertebra on the sacral plateau. This anatomic condition was first described by Herbiniaux, a Belgian obstetrician, in 1782. L5-S1 spondylolisthesis may be acquired or developmental, and usually presents in early childhood. Spondylolisthesis may occur either associated with developmental defects of the anterior or posterior elements (developmental or dysplastic type) or after a spondylolysis, that is, a fracture of the pars interarticularis (acquired or isthmic type). The incidence of unilateral or bilateral pars interarticularis defects is reported to be ~ 4% in children at the age of 6 years, increasing to 6% in adults.[1] Spontaneous healing is almost only in a unilateral pars defect. Bilateral lysis may result in spondylolisthesis because of the mechanical failure of the posterior arch or because of a round sacral dome.

This chapter discusses our current knowledge of the natural history of spondylolisthesis, and reviews the most pertinent classification systems. The discussion of the natural history highlights the role of patient age at diagnosis and the potential worsening of the slippage and deformity throughout life. We also propose a new approach integrating patient age in the characterization and prognostication of spondylolisthesis.

Spondylolisthesis Classifications

The earliest spondylolisthesis classifications described the relationship between L5 vertebra and the sacrum, either the positioning aspects or anatomical aspects. These descriptive aspects were initially presented by the authors as etiological factors, by which they characterized two large families of spondylolisthesis, the isthmic and dysplastic types. More recently, the effect of the pathological relationship between L5 and S1 on the overall spinal alignment was analyzed and resulted in a classification that defines the therapeutic decision and refine the surgical strategy, emphasizing the need for lumbo sacral sagittal realignment. By differentiating low- and high-grade spondylolisthesis, Marchetti and Bartholozzi[2] categorized spondylolisthesis based on the severity of the condition. Later, Hresko and Labelle[3] integrated the recent findings on the spinopelvic balance, and thus were able to move beyond a purely descriptive classification to a more functional analysis. This new approach helped to guide surgical planning based on regional balance. The last version of the Spinal Deformity Study Group (SDSG) classification addresses treatment planning options, however it provides only a snapshot of the spondylolisthesis condition.

Indeed, the grades of spondylolisthesis severity and the occurrence of spinal imbalance describe the progression stages that may occur but may not serve as prognostic factors. Two criteria seem to be of prognostic value: patient age at onset and the presence of a rounded sacrum. We propose a new classification system that addresses both prognosis evaluation and treatment decision-making.

The earliest spondylolisthesis classifications described the relationship between L5 and the sacrum, either the positioning factors or the anatomic factors. These descriptive factors were also considered as etiological factors of the isthmic and dysplastic types of SPL. More recently, the effect of the pathological relationship between L5 and S1 on the overall spinal alignment was analyzed, which resulted in a classification system that addresses management decision making and surgical planning, with an emphasis on the need for lumbosacral sagittal realignment.[4]

Meyerding Grading System

In 1932, Meyerding analyzed the demographic and clinical features of 207 patients presenting at the Mayo Clinic with spondylolisthesis.[5] He proposed a grading system that addresses vertebral slippage based on the degree of subluxation, from grade 1 (25%) to grade 4 (100%). Later, grade 5 was added, representing more than 100% of slippage or spondyloptosis. Meyerding strongly believed that trauma and mechanical overload strains such as obesity, pregnancy, and occupational demands were the main etiologic factors. He also cited the predisposing role of congenital posterior defects that are often associated with this condition. This classification was only descriptive, but it was the first attempt to address the severity of spondylolisthesis displacement.

This first attempt of classification can be criticized as it fails to assess accurately the degree of slippage when the sacrum is round. Indeed, the grading system proposed by Meyerding described a linear displacement of L5 over S1, and it cannot be applied in cases of a round or dome-shaped sacrum.

Segmental Anatomic Classifications: Dysplastic and Isthmic Spondylolisthesis

The classification system that is most often utilized is the one proposed by Wiltse[6] and later modified by Newman, based on the description of the mechanism that produced the spondylolisthesis. The Wiltse classification divided spondylolisthesis into five categories:

I. Dysplastic
II. Isthmic
    a. Spondylolysis
    b. Isthmus elongation
    c. Acute fracture
III. Traumatic
IV. Degenerative
V. Pathological

According to this classification, the most frequent types in children and adolescents are the dysplastic (type I) and the isthmic types (type II).

Type I is associated with congenital dysplasia of L5 or S1. Fredrickson et al[1] found a high frequency of spina occulta and S1 dysplastic changes associated with spondylolisthesis. The congenital anomalies of the posterior elements were recognized as key factors for the occurrence of progressive slippage. Fredrickson et al and later Beutler et al[7] described the frequency of progression based on the associated abnormalities. Lonstein[8] also compared these two types, and suggested that sacral doming was a congenital defect due to an anterior growth disturbance and was the main factor contributing to lumbosacral kyphosis.

Wiltse did not address the role of anterior dysplastic changes in the progression of spondylolisthesis. (We will discuss the importance of these changes later in the chapter.) Moreover, Wiltse did not differentiate pars elongation from true spondylolisthesis produced by the slippage of L5. This differentiation seems to us to be of clinical and therapeutical relevance, as closed spondylolisthesis with progressive sliding will progressively reduce the size of the canal and consequently induce spinal stenosis.

In the isthmic type, the pars interarticularis is disrupted, first stage being spondylolysis (pars fracture without slippage). The most common mechanism is an acquired fatigue fracture. Wiltse et al[6] and later Fredrickson et al[1] demonstrated that spondylolysis was produced after the acquisition of bipedalism. The incidence of SPL increases during growth, from 5% at 7 years to 7% at skeletal maturity.[1,6] Wiltse suggested three subgroups based on the healing process: -spondylolytic stress fracture without signs of healing (fibrous tissue is seen surrounding the pars defect), -pars elongation (the healing process occurs on a dysplastic posterior arch), -acute traumatic fracture (which also could be included in type III). Pars elongation could also be included in the dysplastic type (type I), which is always associated with congenital dysplasia of the L5 or S1 posterior arches.

In 1997, Marchetti and Bartholozzi[2] proposed a new classification distinguishing developmental from acquired spondylolisthesis. In developmental spondylolisthesis, they defined two subgroups—low grade and high grade—based on the importance of the dysplastic changes. In low-grade dysplastic spondylolisthesis, the sacral plateau remains flat and L5 remains rectangular. High-grade dysplastic spondylolisthesis is characterized by a dome-shaped sacral end plate and a trapezoidal L5 vertebral body. The authors intended this classification to guide the management of spondylolisthesis patients, based on the risk of progression of the dysplastic changes.

Even though this classification may help in the management of high-grade dysplastic spondylolisthesis, it does not clarify either the spectrum of situations requiring surgical management or the decision of whether to fuse in situ or to perform surgical reduction.

The acquired spondylolisthesis group includes traumatic, iatrogenic, pathological, and degenerative spondylolisthesis related to an excessive loading stress applied to the pars interarticularis. Again, this classification does not help to determine the treatment strategy for stabilizing and normalizing spinal morphology and restoring spinal balance, even if it highlights some of the prognostic factors leading to spondylolisthesis aggravation process.

Neither the Wiltse nor the Marchetti-Bartholozzi classification was designed to guide decision making for spondylolisthesis treatment. It was not until the era of sagittal balance understanding, that the slippage phenomenon was integrated into the global spinal balance, helping to provide some critical therapeutic recommendations.

Global Anatomic Classification

New classifications integrating the pathological relationship between L5 and the sacrum into the overall context of spinal balance arose in the early 21st century, in order to differentiate balanced versus unbalanced situations. Once the spondylolisthesis has destabilized spinal balance, surgical management requires both a reduction strategy and stabilization.

During et al[9] were the first group to link the lumbosacral postural parameters. They described the pelvisacral angle, which is the complement angle to pelvic incidence (PI). In their original work, they were also the first to report a significant difference of the spino pelvic angles between spondylolisthesis patients and controls.[9]

In 2004, Labelle and Roussouly's group[10] found that specific pelvic shapes were associated with spondylolisthesis and that PI was correlated with the degree of slippage, suggesting that a high PI was a risk factor for spondylolisthesis. Later, some authors, such as Huang et al[11] and Whitesides et al,[12] criticized the prognostic value of PI. Roussouly et al,[13] therefore, differentiated two types of pelvic orientation that may produce spondylolisthesis by different mechanism: the shear type and the nutcracker type.

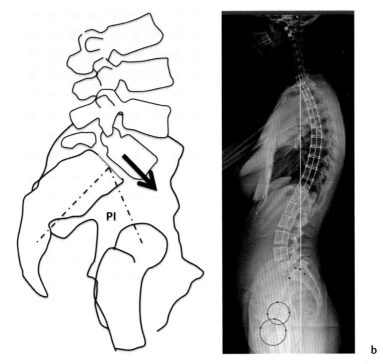

a   b

Fig. 10.1 **(a)** In high pelvic incidence (PI), the corresponding high sacral slope (SS) induces shear forces and L5 slippage. **(b)** A radiograph of a patient with painful L5 lysis, with PI = 78 degrees and SS = 58 degrees.

The shear type is characterized by a high PI, which increases the shear stress on the L5-S1 level due to a high sacral slope (**Fig. 10.1**). More than 70% of lumbar lordosis is expressed in the lower arc of lordosis (L4–S1), which is generally equal to the sacral slope. Inoue et al[14] further confirmed the prognostic value of the morphology and orientation of the sacrum, emphasizing the importance of the shape of the sacral plateau. They also described the sacral table angle (STA), the angle between the sacral end plate and the posterior aspect of S1, and showed that in children and adolescents with L5-S1 spondylolisthesis the anatomy of the sacrum was different from that in the general population.

The nutcracker type is associated with a low PI. Spondylolysis is produced by the direct compression forces exerted by the L4 inferior facets on the L5 pars interarticularis. The association with a type 1 sagittal morphology (in the Roussouly classification[15]) increases the constraints, as the lumbar lordosis is low and

is mainly expressed at the L4, L5, and S1 levels (**Fig. 10.2**).[16]

In 2007, Hresko et al[3] proposed a new classification system integrating both the slippage grade and the sagittal spinopelvic balance. This new classification system evaluates progression, and addresses the treatment of decision making spondylolisthesis. The chief goal of this new classification was to integrate the contributions of previous classification systems, especially that of Bartholozzi and Marchetti, as well as the concept of spinopelvic balance, which is important in understanding human spinal pathology. With improved understanding of sagittal alignment and analysis of spinopelvic parameters, the factors of spinal balance and imbalance are now well characterized. Hresko et al identified two subgroups of patients with high-grade spondylolisthesis, based on whether the pelvis was balanced or unbalanced (**Fig. 10.3**)—low-grade spondylolisthesis being also balanced. The pelvic tilt and sacral slope values were similar between controls and the balanced

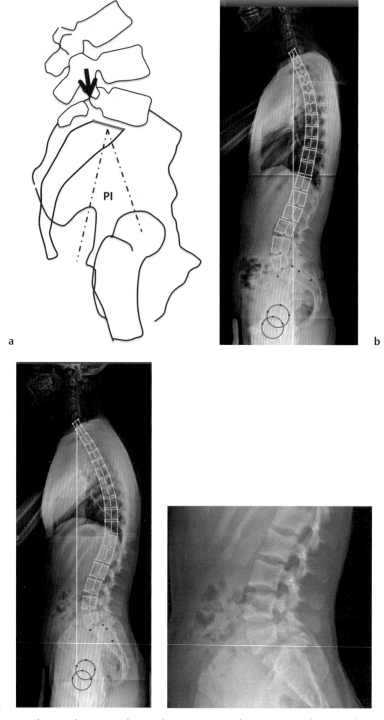

Fig. 10.2 **(a)** Nutcracker mechanism: in low PI the distal hyperlordosis induces L4-L5 hyperextension. L5 isthmic breakage is due to L4 facet impaction. **(b)** A radiograph of an 18-year-old man with type 1 pelvic orientation in Roussouly's classification.

PI = 48 degrees. Note the L4-L5 hyperextension. **(c)** A radiograph of a 20-year-old man with low back pain. The PI is 37 degrees, which is very low. Multilevel isthmic lysis (L3, L4, L5) is seen, with a type 1 profile.

Balanced **Retroverted**

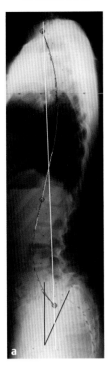
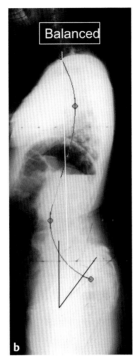
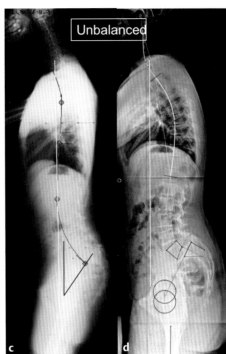

Fig. 10.3 Radiographs demonstrating Hresko's classification. **(a,b)** Radiographs of a well-balanced patient with no pelvic retroversion. The C7 plumb line is behind the femoral heads. **(c)** A radiograph of a retroverted balanced patient with increasing pelvic tilt (PT) and hyperlordosis of the lumbar region. The goal is to maintain the C7 plumb line behind the femoral heads. **(d)** Radiograph of a retroverted unbalanced patient with high PT and high lumbar lordosis. The C7 plumb line behind the femoral heads could not be maintained.

pelvis patients. Unbalanced pelvis (retroverted) patients had a sagittal spinal alignment that differed from the balanced pelvis patients and the control group, suggesting that reduction techniques might be considered in patients with an unbalanced pelvis. In these patients, the importance of slippage was related to the following regional modifications: sacral doming, trapezoidal L5 vertebra, lumbosacral kyphosis (described by Dubousset[17]) and increased L5 incidence.[18]

However, this classification could only describe the consequences of high-grade spondylolisthesis based on the importance of sacral morphology modifications. But it is important also to address the sliding-mechanism concept that produces the L5-S1 spondylolisthe-sis. Indeed, the existence of a sacral dome, in association with dysplasia of the posterior elements, causes a rotational displacement of the L5 vertebral body on S1, from the moment when the mechanical failure occurs (**Fig. 10.4**).

Spinal Deformity Study Group Classification

Labelle et al[19] and the SDSG, an international group of spinal surgeons, implemented a clinical and radiological prospective database with low- and high-grade SPL patients. From these data, the SDSG tried to simplify this synthetic approach, classifying progression into six types (**Fig. 10.5**). This classification system initially intended to assess the slippage grade, the

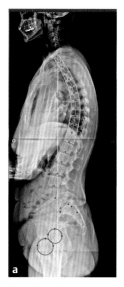
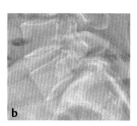
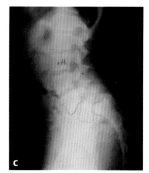
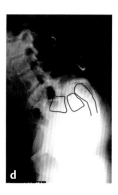

Fig. 10.4 The evolution of L5 isthmic lysis in an adult. **(a)** A radiograph of a patient with longitudinal sliding on a flat sacrum linked to the progressive collapsing of the L5-S1 degenerative disk. **(b)** Close-up view of lumbosacral region demonstrating parallel olisthesis of L5 on S1. **(c,d)** Radiographs of a patient with a round course of L5 around the dome-shaped sacral end. **(c)** At the age of 14 years, the patient is grade 3 and grade 4. **(d)** At the age of 40 years, the patient has complete ptosis with severe unbalance.

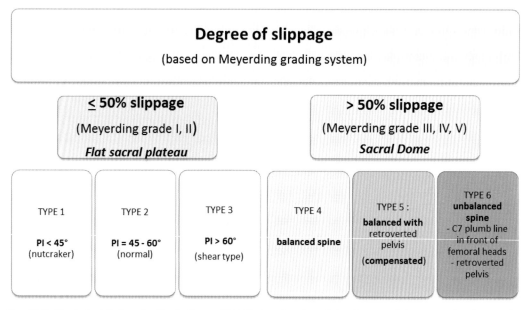

Fig. 10.5 The Spinal Deformity Study Group (SDSG) classification of the degree of slippage in lumbosacral spondylolisthesis, based on the Meyerding grading system. PI, pelvic incidence.

degree of dysplasia, and the sacropelvic sagittal balance, but to simplify the reliability testing, the assessment of dysplasia was excluded.[20]

In the subgroup of spondylolysis and low-grade spondylolisthesis with less than 50% slippage (Wiltse grade 0, 1, or 2), we can define three types based on the pelvic morphology. This subgroup includes the two etiologic categories defined by Roussouly (nutcracker and shear types). The intermediate group, type 2, mainly includes dysplastic spondylolisthesis.

The high-grade spondylolisthesis group is classified based on the sagittal spinopelvic balance. The spine can either be balanced with low pelvic tilt, which may require in situ fusion, or unbalanced with a lumbosacral kyphosis inducing pelvic retroversion. Anterior translation of the spine above the sacrum induces positional compensations to maintain the projection of the gravity line above the hips. When compensatory mechanisms are insufficient, the C7 plumb line falls forward in the hip axis. There is no specific health-related quality-of-life questionnaire that addresses spondylolisthesis. However, Harroud et al[21] found a clear correlation between sagittal malalignment in untreated high-grade spondylolisthesis patients and scores on the Scoliosis Research Society Outcomes Questionnaire (SRS-22) in all domains—except the mental health score. The MICD (Minimal Clinically Important Difference) was reached for the unbalanced type (C7 plumb line in front of the hip axis), especially on the pain and appearance domains.[21] Therefore, reduction and fusion are addressed to achieve an optimal result in type 5 and 6 patients[21] (**Table 10.1**).

A purely anatomic description of the slippage of L5 on S1 and of the anomalies of the posterior arch has resulted in an analysis of the anatomic region, including the balance and spinal functions. Although the SDSG classification describes all the stages of progression of spondylolisthesis and addresses the pelvic morphology and the sagittal sacropelvic balance, it provides only a snapshot of the current situation and does not predict the natural history and the risk of progression. The main objectives of a classification of L5-S1 spondylolisthesis are to assess the risk of progression and to help determine the optimal treatment strategy. The major drawback of the latest SDSG classification is that it does not address patient age, and thus it fails to assess the remaining spinal growth potential and to predict the degenerative changes in adulthood.

Natural History: Proposal for a New Classification Integrating the Dimension of Age

In a previous classification, Marchetti and Bartholozzi attempted to address the variable of patient age, without which the prognostic factors for progression of spondylolisthesis could not be determined.

The risk of progression in children and adolescents is dependent on many mechanical and developmental factors as well as on the degeneration that comes with aging. The different classification systems have all contributed in various ways to the goal of providing a complete picture of the spondylolisthesis. Now all these systems must be synthesized to assess

Table 10.1 Proposed Surgical Treatment Strategy Based on the Hresko Classification

Sacropelvic Alignment	Spinopelvic Balance	Surgical Strategy
Normal	Balanced	In situ fusion
Retroverted	Balanced	360-degree fusion; discuss the possibility of performing reduction
	Unbalanced (C7 plumb line is in front of the femoral heads)	360-degree fusion; reduction is mandatory

this disease throughout a patient's lifetime. For example, a grade IV slippage later in life may have been grade I at an earlier age; L5 slippage is a major component of the deformity, and it is strongly correlated with the severity of the disease.[20] As another example, lumbosacral kyphosis is strongly correlated with quality of life.[21,22] Thus, these two factors, slippage and lumbosacral kyphosis, are consequences of disease progression rather than risk factors.

The goal of a new classification is to integrate the various features described above in one classification that addresses both descriptive (anatomic) factors and prognostic factors of the disease across the patient's lifetime.

Three major elements should be taken into account:

1. Local anatomic abnormalities, such as posterior arch dysplasia and a sacral dome
2. Spinopelvic parameters, such as pelvic incidence (PI), pelvic tilt (PT), lumbar lordosis (LL), L5 slippage and the presence of reciprocal spinal curvatures in the pelvis
3. Patient age at diagnosis and related factors, such as the remaining skeletal growth potential, the mechanical impact, and the associated degeneration

The amount of slippage is the direct consequence of spondylolisthesis progression but is not a prognostic factor in itself. We propose to assess the natural history of spondylolisthesis in relation to the patient's age and initial status (e.g., dysplastic, isthmic lysis) and at the time of diagnosis.

Dysplastic Spondylolisthesis: Development-Associated Abnormalities

Marchetti and Bartholozzi[2] have addressed the role of dysplasia in the progression of spondylolisthesis. The wedging of the L5 vertebra (trapezoidal aspect of the vertebral body) evaluated by the Taillard index or the height ratio between the anterior and posterior walls has been shown to be a risk factor for progres-

sion. Similarly, a convex sacral plate may be present prior to slippage and may increase the shear stress on the L5-S1 level.

Most authors agree that slippage is responsible for the secondary deformity of the L5 vertebral body and sacral doming. However, Terai et al[23] and Gutman et al[24] reported an early stable L5-S1 spondylolisthesis with formation of a dome before the growth spurt, and total reconstruction of the sacral plateau, aligned with L5, at the end of the growth spurt. Gutman et al suggested that the dome production could be associated with a dystrophic mechanism comparable to Scheuermann disease (**Fig. 10.6**).[24] A dome-shaped sacrum is a secondary process related to the mechanical constraints that disturb the ossification of the sacral end plate during growth. Sacral doming may also occur in low-grade spondylolisthesis and may be explained by genetically driven risk factors for dystrophic changes of the vertebral end plates, as seen in Scheuermann kyphosis.

Dome shaping of the sacral end plate is highly correlated with high-grade spondylolisthesis, with higher slippage and a greater risk of lumbosacral kyphosis (unbalanced spine) than with the flat sacrum type. This could be explained by the progression of L5 slippage at the rounded end of the sacrum. This progression also induces tilting of L5, increasing the L5 incidence, as well as lumbosacral kyphosis. Analysis of untreated adults with a dysplastic high-grade spondylolisthesis demonstrates a continuous impairment of grading, leading to total ptosis and a highly unbalanced condition.

Isthmic Spondylolysis: Role of the Pelvic Shape

Numerous L5 isthmic lyses occur with a flat sacral plateau after the growth spurt. It is generally difficult to differentiate a preexisting lysis from a recent stress fracture of the L5 isthmus. In contrast to a dome-shaped sacrum, L5 lysis with flat sacral plateau facilitates calculating the PI.

Pelvic incidence is the pelvic morphological angle, defined as the angle between the perpendicular line to the sacral plate and the line

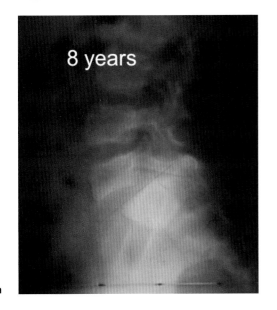

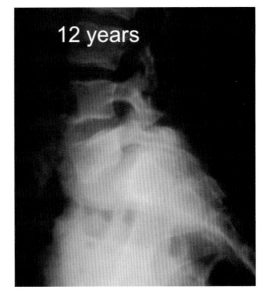

a

b

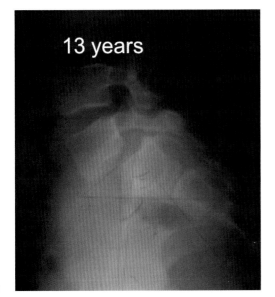

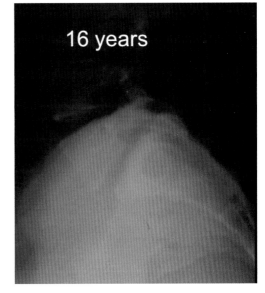

d

Fig. 10.6 (a) Initial radiograph of a stable pars elongation of L5 with grade 2 spondylolisthesis. **(b–d)** The progressive appearance of a dome during growth, with total reconstruction of the sacral end when full growth is achieved.

joining the middle of the sacral plate and the center of the femoral heads. This angle is constant in adulthood but has been shown to increase during growth.[25,26] Labelle et al[10] found that the PI, SS, and LL are significantly greater in patients with spondylolisthesis as compared with controls. They reported an average PI value of 63 degrees in spondylolisthesis patients, while PI averaged 52 degrees in an asymptomatic population. Due to a strong correlation between PI and SS, the higher the PI, the higher the SS. This higher PI may explain a shear stress mechanism that is related to the increased SS. Labelle et al also found that the risk of higher slippage was correlated with a higher PI.[10] This increasing slippage generally occurs in adults with L5-S1 disc degeneration, as if the loss of the disc height facilitates increasing slippage.

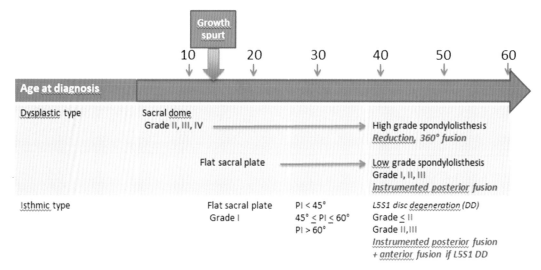

Fig. 10.7 A proposed new classification system that addresses the sliding mechanism. This classification is prognostic, not just descriptive, as it assesses the growth dimension. It provides recommendations for the management of spondylolisthesis, based on patient age at the time of diagnosis and on the existing risk factors (such as a sacral dome, a high PI, or a type 4 curve). It assesses the risk of progression of the slippage, and therefore the occurrence of compensation mechanisms in cases of spinal imbalance. The first scenario in this classification is characterized by a flat sacrum. The risk of progression and the therapeutic recommendations depend on the spinopelvic parameters and the dysplastic changes of the posterior arch. There is a risk of progression in case of a highly dysplastic lumbosacral junction with a low PI, but the spondylolisthesis remains low grade, whereas patients with high PI may have high-grade spondylolisthesis, especially when associated with dysplasia and L5S1 disc degeneration. If L5S1 disc degenerates, spondylolisthesis may aggravate, but only in a translational mode (low grade spondylolisthesis). Second scenario is characterized by a dome-shaped sacrum, in which the PI cannot be measured. Dome-shaped sacrum can only occur before the growth spurt. The risk of progression is high. The slippage mechanism is situated around the dome and is associated with a much higher rate of lumbar lordosis progression and lumbosacral kyphosis. Patients in this group are at higher risk of sagittal imbalance because of lumbosacral kyphosis.

L5 slippage never surpasses 50% (Meyerding grade II), as it is limited by the tension of the anterior ligament, even once the L5-S1 disc has totally collapsed. Translational L5 slippage may have the following consequences:

- Local instability
- L5 nerve root by foraminal compression or traction
- Spinopelvic sagittal imbalancein high-grade spondylolisthesis (> 50% slippage)

Due to the rarity of low PI in spondylolisthesis patients, Roussouly's group[15] described a specific situation in a patient with low PI and a type 1 back shape, characterized by a long thoracolumbar kyphosis and a short lumbar hyperlordosis.[15] This local hyperextension, mainly expressed at levels L4-L5 and L5-S1, induces a stress impact of the L4 inferior facet on the L5 isthmus, causing an acquired stress fracture. The structural and distal hyperextension of the lumbar spine produces pain because of the nutcracker mechanism. The stress on the L5-S1 disc may lead to early degeneration, which increases the slippage. A thoracolumbar kyphosis induced by Scheuermann disease may increase the severity of the mechanical process.

Thus, the proposed new classification addresses the natural history of L5-S1 spondylolisthesis as related to patient age at diagnosis (**Fig. 10.7**). This classification is prognostic, not just descriptive, as it includes assessment of the growth dimension. It helps to determine the appropriate treatment based on patient age at the time of diagnosis as well as on the risk factors (such as a sacral dome, a high PI, a type 4 curve), yielding an accurate description of the risk of spondylolisthesis progression, even in low grade spondylolisthesis, and of the occurrence of compensatory mechanisms in case of spinal imbalance.

Two important periods may be differentiated and may define two types of spondylolisthesis natural history: childhood until the growth spurt and adulthood (the degenerative process related to aging process). In case of isthmic elongation or spondylolysis occurring before the growth spurt, the risk of developing a dome shape is high and is generally producing high-grade spondylolisthesis. Permanent slippage may lead to a complete vertebral ptosis in adulthood. In patients with isthmic lysis and a flat sacral plateau, there is absolutely no risk of the dome shape if spondylolysis occurs after the growth spurt. In these patients, the PI may be accurately measured, and it is an excellent indicator of the etiologic mechanism of SPL and its prognosis. If the PI is low (< 45 degrees), the pathophysiological mechanism is the nutcracker phenomenon, which entails a painful evolution and the risk of slippage. When the PI is in the normal range (45 to 65 degrees), the spondylolisthesis is well balanced and moderately painful, but the risk of slippage in adulthood remains in case of L5-S1 disc degeneration. With higher values of PI (> 65 degrees), due to the increasing SS and the shear stress on the intervertebral disc, spondylolisthesis is more unstable and may generate chronic low back pain, necessitating early surgery. In adulthood the risk of slippage depending on L5S1 disc degeneration, and may produce and worsen spinal imbalance. However L5 slippage will never exceed 50%.

⫶ Chapter Summary

The three main classification systems that have been used for L5-S1 spondylolisthesis are able to determine the importance of L5 slippage,

the anatomy of the L5 posterior arch, the level of dysplasia, and the effect of L5-S1 misplacement on the global sagittal spinal balance. But none of these classifications predicts the risk of progression of L5-S1 spondylolisthesis. Depending on the combination of the various risk factors, the occurrence of vertebral slippage can vary in frequency and is age dependent, based on the remaining growth potential. The role of anterior vertebral dysplasia (existence of a sacral dome, wedging of L5) is of particular importance, as it increases the sacral slope and lowers the sliding resistance.

A dome-shaped sacrum only occurs before the growth spurt, which is a key period in the patient's life cycle; after the growth spurt, a sacral plateau that is flat will remain so. If the dome-shaped sacrum entails the risk of permanent slippage in adulthood, then the flat sacrum's degenerative progression is determined by the SS orientation and consequently by the PI angle.

Pearls

◆ Determine if the sacral end is dome shaped or flat.
◆ Determine the PI only at the flat sacral end and in a dome with an L5 tilt (L5 incidence and lumbo sacral angle (LSA)).
◆ Sagittal balance is affected by the L5 tilt rather than by the L5 slippage.
◆ It is important to determine the appearance of the dome during the growth spurt in children.
◆ In adults, L5-S1 disk degeneration causes longitudinal slippage in a flat sacrum. The dome undergoes continuous rounding slippage of L5, which can lead to total ptosis.

Pitfalls

◆ Do not fail to measure the PI in the dome-shaped sacrum.
◆ Do not ignore sagittal balance when planning surgery and deciding between in situ fusion or reduction.
◆ Differentiate pathophisiological mechanisms: shear stress or nutcracker mechanism.
◆ Do not ignore the PI value in patients with L5 isthmic lysis and a flat sacrum.

References

Five Must-Read References

1. Fredrickson BE, Baker D, McHolick WJ, Yuan HA, Lubicky JP. The natural history of spondylolysis and spondylolisthesis. J Bone Joint Surg Am 1984;66:699–707

2. Marchetti PG, Bartholozzi P. Classification of spondylolisthesis as a guideline for treatment. In: Bridwell KH, DeWald RL, eds. Textbook of Spinal Surgery, 2nd ed. Philadelphia: Lippincott-Raven; 1997:1211–1254

3. Hresko MT, Labelle H, Roussouly P, Berthonnaud E. Classification of high-grade spondylolistheses based on pelvic version and spine balance: possible rationale for reduction. Spine 2007;32:2208–2213

4. Mac-Thiong J-M, Duong L, Parent S, et al. Reliability of the Spinal Deformity Study Group classification of lumbosacral spondylolisthesis. Spine 2012;37:E95–E102

5. Wright IP. Who was Meyerding? Spine 2003;28:733–735

6. Wiltse LL, Newman PH, Macnab I. Classification of spondylolisis and spondylolisthesis. Clin Orthop Relat Res 1976;117:23–29

7. Beutler WJ, Fredrickson BE, Murtland A, Sweeney CA, Grant WD, Baker D. The natural history of spondylolysis and spondylolisthesis: 45-year follow-up evaluation. Spine 2003;28:1027–1035, discussion 1035

8. Lonstein JE. Spondylolisthesis in children. Cause, natural history, and management. Spine 1999;24:2640–2648

9. During J, Goudfrooij H, Keessen W, Beeker TW, Crowe A. Toward standards for posture. Postural characteristics of the lower back system in normal and pathologic conditions. Spine 1985;10:83–87

10. Labelle H, Roussouly P, Berthonnaud E, et al. Spondylolisthesis, pelvic incidence, and spinopelvic balance: a correlation study. Spine 2004;29:2049–2054

11. Huang RP, Bohlman HH, Thompson GH, Poe-Kochert C. Predictive value of pelvic incidence in progression of spondylolisthesis. Spine 2003;28:2381–2385, discussion 2385

12. Whitesides TE Jr, Horton WC, Hutton WC, Hodges L. Spondylolytic spondylolisthesis: a study of pelvic and lumbosacral parameters of possible etiologic effect in two genetically and geographically distinct groups with high occurrence. Spine 2005; 30(6, Suppl):S12–S21

13. Roussouly P, Gollogly S, Berthonnaud E, Labelle H, Weidenbaum M. Sagittal alignment of the spine and pelvis in the presence of L5-S1 isthmic lysis and low-grade spondylolisthesis. Spine 2006;31:2484–2490

14. Inoue H, Ohmori K, Miyasaka K. Radiographic classification of L5 isthmic spondylolisthesis as adolescent or adult vertebral slip. Spine 2002;27:831–838

15. Vaz G, Roussouly P, Berthonnaud E, Dimnet J. Sagittal morphology and equilibrium of pelvis and spine. Eur Spine J 2002;11:80–87

16. Roussouly P, Pinheiro-Franco JL. Biomechanical analysis of the spino-pelvic organization and adaptation in pathology. Eur Spine J 2011;20(Suppl 5):609–618

17. Dubousset J. Treatment of spondylolysis and spondylolisthesis in children and adolescents. Clin Orthop Relat Res 1997;337:77–85

18. Labelle H, Roussouly P, Berthonnaud E, Dimnet J, O'Brien M. The importance of spino-pelvic balance in L5-s1 developmental spondylolisthesis: a review of pertinent radiologic measurements. Spine 2005;

19. Labelle H, Mac-Thiong J-M, Roussouly P. Spino-pelvic sagittal balance of spondylolisthesis: a review and classification. Eur Spine J 2011;20(Suppl 5):641–646

20. Mac-Thiong J-M, Labelle H, Parent S, Hresko MT, Deviren V, Weidenbaum M; members of the Spinal Deformity Study Group. Reliability and development of a new classification of lumbosacral spondylolisthesis. Scoliosis 2008;3:19

21. Harroud A, Labelle H, Joncas J, Mac-Thiong J-M. Global sagittal alignment and health-related quality of life in lumbosacral spondylolisthesis. Eur Spine J 2013;22:849–856

22. Tanguay F, Labelle H, Wang Z, Joncas J, de Guise JA, Mac-Thiong J-M. Clinical significance of lumbosacral kyphosis in adolescent spondylolisthesis. Spine 2012;37:304–308

23. Terai T, Sairyo K, Goel VK, et al. Biomechanical rationale of sacral rounding deformity in pediatric spondylolisthesis: a clinical and biomechanical study. Arch Orthop Trauma Surg 2011;131:1187–1194

24. Gutman G, Silvestre C, Roussouly P. Sacral doming progression in developmental spondylolisthesis: a demonstrative case report with two different evolutions. Eur Spine J 2014;23(Suppl 2):288–295

25. Abelin-Genevois K, Idjerouidene A, Roussouly P, Vital JM, Garin C. Cervical spine alignment in the pediatric population: a radiographic normative study of 150 asymptomatic patients. Eur Spine J 2014;23:1442–1448

26. Mac-Thiong J-M, Labelle H, Roussouly P. Pediatric sagittal alignment. Eur Spine J 2011;20(Suppl 5):586–590

Adolescent Spondylolisthesis Associated with Scoliosis: Which Condition Should Surgery Address?

Yong Qiu

Introduction

Spondylolisthesis is the common cause of low back pain in adolescents.[1] The incidence of scoliosis in patients with spondylolysis or spondylolisthesis has been well reported in the literature, with the percentage ranging from 15% to 48%.[2,3] Conversely, the incidence of spondylolisthesis in idiopathic scoliosis patients was documented to be 6.2%,[3] which is appreciably higher than that found in the general population, ranging from 4.4% at the age of 6 years to 6% in adulthood.[4] Most of the existing investigations focused on the relationship between adult scoliosis and lumbar degenerative spondylolisthesis, whereas only a few studies reported the association of scoliosis with spondylolisthesis in the adolescent population.[2,3,5–7] As highlighted in the literature, the true incidence of the two deformities occurring concomitantly in one patient is difficult to determine, and there is no consensus on the optimal management strategy.[6,8,9] This chapter discusses how spondylolisthesis associated with scoliosis influences decision making in the treatment of adolescent patients.

Etiology of Scoliosis Associated with Spondylolisthesis

Fisk et al[3] were the first to conduct a study on scoliosis associated with spondylolisthesis in adolescents. They found that 48% of the patients with spondylolisthesis had concomitant scoliosis. Several studies[6,7,10,11] focusing on adolescent scoliosis associated with spondylolisthesis were then performed, and scoliosis associated with spondylolisthesis has been divided into three main categories[5]:

Type I: idiopathic scoliosis in the upper spine (thoracic or thoracolumbar curve), which is not considered to be related to the olisthetic defect (**Fig. 11.1**)

Type II: scoliosis resulting from the olisthetic defect and rotational displacement of the lumbar vertebra in relation to the sacrum (**Fig. 11.2**)

Type III: "sciatic" scoliosis, which is considered secondary to nerve root compression and muscle spasm induced by spondylolisthesis (**Fig. 11.3**)

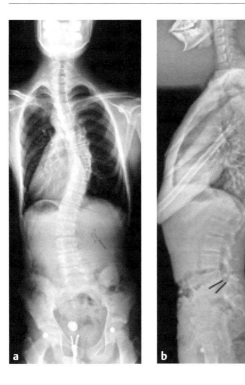

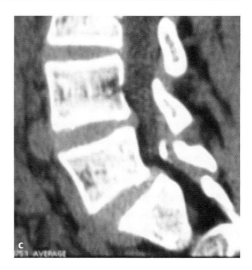

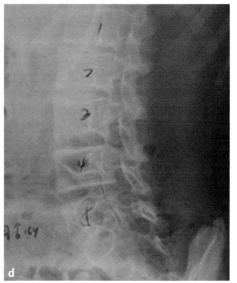

Fig. 11.1 Radiographs of a 16-year-old boy with **(a,b)** idiopathic thoracic scoliosis associated with **(c,d)** grade I isthmic spondylolisthesis at L5-S1.

In type I, idiopathic scoliosis with concomitant spondylolisthesis, patients usually have a typical thoracic or thoracolumbar curve and a positive family history.[3] They usually present initially with scoliosis because of their cosmetic concerns; they are otherwise asymptomatic.[3,12] They typically have a right thoracic curve or a left lumbar curve, with a well-balanced spine.[6,13] Generally, the spondylolisthesis is an accidental finding on radiography. It is generally believed that the two pathologies are not dependent on each other.[6] However, some authors suggest that thoracolumbar or lumbar idiopathic scoliosis can induce spondylolysis because of asymmetrical stress and strain during the growth period.[11] I believe that the lumbar idiopathic curve should be considered as an independent spinal deformity, if it complies with the features mentioned above and if the apical lumbar vertebral rotation is larger than that of the slipped vertebra. Based on these criteria, it would be reasonable to conclude that idiopathic scoliosis and spondylolisthesis occur independently in these patients and neither one affects the occurrence of the other (**Fig. 11.1**).

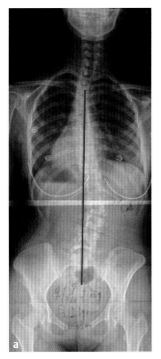
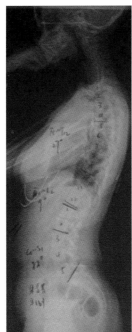
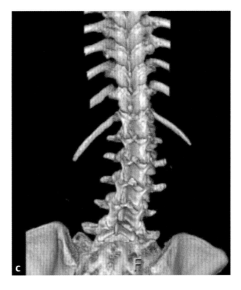
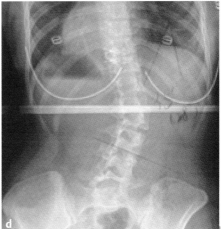

Fig. 11.2 Radiographs of a 16-year-old girl with **(a,b)** scoliosis associated with grade I isthmic spondylolisthesis at L5-S1. **(c)** Computed tomography (CT) scans showed an L5 bilateral spondylolysis and an L5 rotation (13 degrees). **(d)** Anteroposterior (AP) lumbar spine radiograph showed rotation of the L5 pedicles.

In type II, scoliosis resulting from an olisthetic defect, several features distinguish patients from those with an idiopathic scoliosis. The curve associated with an asymmetric olisthetic defect is usually more rotated than an idiopathic scoliosis curve that is of a similar severity.[13] Unlike idiopathic scoliosis, in which the apical vertebra rotates the most, the spondylolytic vertebra has the maximal rotation in scoliosis secondary to an olisthetic defect.[13,14] A possible mechanism is that the asymmetric olisthesis creates an asymmetric foundation, which may cause the upper spine to rotate into a torsional lumbar scoliosis (**Fig. 11.2**). The etio-

pathogenesis was first explained by Tojner.[14] According to his theory, in a spine with bilateral spondylolysis, the lytic vertebra may slip and rotate on the narrower spondylolisthesis gap. Then the rotation can cause the lateral shift of the olisthetic vertebra and exert traction on the intervertebral disk, especially on the side opposite the axis of rotation, leading to vertebral body sinking on that side. This "sinking" of an olisthetic vertebral body can create an asymmetric foundation of the upper spine, and can further induce the loss of static balance and the development of a compensatory scoliosis. However, there are several controversies about

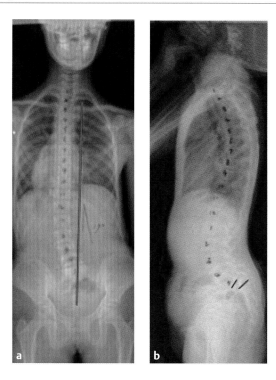
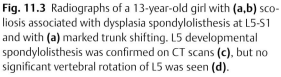
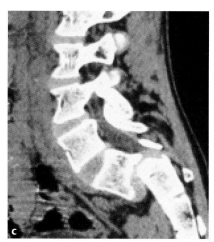
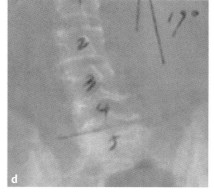

Fig. 11.3 Radiographs of a 13-year-old girl with **(a,b)** scoliosis associated with dysplasia spondylolisthesis at L5-S1 and with **(a)** marked trunk shifting. L5 developmental spondylolisthesis was confirmed on CT scans **(c)**, but no significant vertebral rotation of L5 was seen **(d)**.

this theory. Schlenzka[15] questioned whether the rotational slip was the first event leading to the development of a scoliosis above the vertebra, or whether the rotation of the spondylolytic vertebra developed secondarily as in an ordinary idiopathic lumbar curve. In particular, unlike "sciatic" scoliosis, olisthetic scoliosis usually has no coronal shifting (**Fig. 11.2**). In short, "olisthetic" scoliosis usually presents with an asymmetric olisthetic defect (unstable asymmetric foundation and torsion scoliosis), and the maximum rotation occurs at the olisthetic defect rather than at the curve apex. These patients may complain of leg pain.

Type III, "sciatic" scoliosis, is characterized by coronal decompensation caused by foraminal nerve root compression and muscle spasm in patients with symptomatic spondylolisthesis. Sciatic scoliosis is a functional (nonstructural) secondary deformity and is usually characterized by having little or no vertebral rotation, hamstring tightness, and coronal imbalance (thoracic trunk shift). This is similar to lumbar scoliosis caused by nerve root compression and muscle spasm in other spine diseases (e.g., lumbar disk herniation, osteoid osteoma) (**Fig. 11.3**). The clinical features of sciatic scoliosis are as follows: (1) low back pain as the presenting complaint; (2) trunk shifting with a small curve angle but a long curve span; and (3) back muscle spasm as an additional presenting complaint.

In my center, 30 cases of adolescent spondylolisthesis were treated surgically between 2002 and 2014. Of these patients, 14 (46.7%) had concomitant scoliosis, of whom eight patients were diagnosed as spondylolisthesis-associated adolescent idiopathic scoliosis (AIS) (type I).

Natural History of Scoliosis Associated with Spondylolisthesis

It is difficult to explain why in some cases a slipped vertebra, which is intrinsically unstable, does not lead to the occurrence of scoliosis, whereas in other cases the slipped vertebra triggers the development not only of scoliosis but also of curve progression. In adolescent scoliosis associated with spondylolisthesis, it is possible that the curve evolves together with the increase of the spondylolisthesis during the growth spurts. As a case example, a 12-year-old girl complained of low back pain (**Fig. 11.4**).

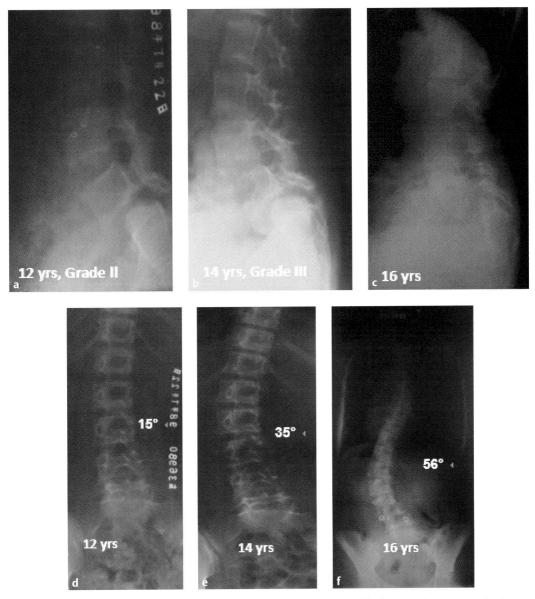

Fig. 11.4 Radiographs of a 12-year-old girl with **(a,d)** scoliosis associated with dysplastic spondylolisthesis. **(b,e)** The spondylolisthesis upgraded to grade III, and scoliosis progressed to 35 degrees. **(c,f)** The spondylolisthesis and curve magnitude increased to grade IV and 56 degrees, respectively, at the age of 16. (*continued on page 104*)

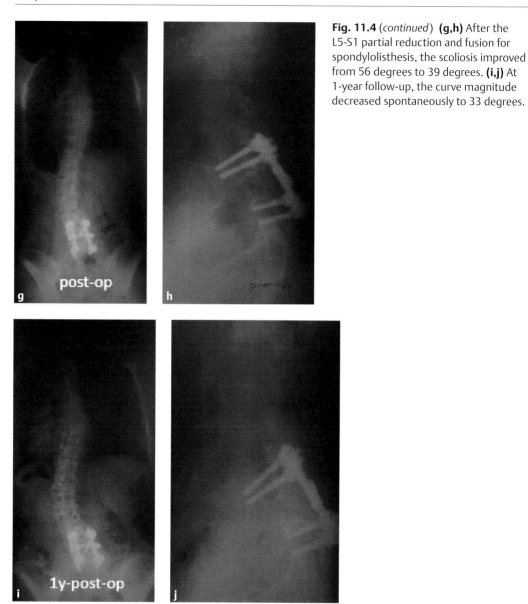

Fig. 11.4 (*continued*) **(g,h)** After the L5-S1 partial reduction and fusion for spondylolisthesis, the scoliosis improved from 56 degrees to 39 degrees. **(i,j)** At 1-year follow-up, the curve magnitude decreased spontaneously to 33 degrees.

Anteroposterior radiographs demonstrated a grade II dysplastic spondylolisthesis at L5-S1 associated with a lumbar curve of 15 degrees. The spondylolisthesis increased from grade II to grade IV, and concomitantly the scoliosis progressed to 56 degrees during the next 4 years. As the scoliosis and vertebral rotation evolved with the progression of spondylolisthesis, we can speculate that the occurrence and deterioration of scoliosis could be attributed to progressive spondylolisthesis.

▪ Treatment Principles in Adolescent Spondylolisthesis Associated with Scoliosis

For AIS with spondylolisthesis, it is believed that the two pathologies should be managed separately using the generally accepted treatment methods for each condition.[2,3,5,13] For asymptomatic spondylolysis with mild idiopathic scoliosis, conservative treatment for the scoliosis, such as observation or bracing, is recommended.[3] If the curve progresses to more than 45 to 50 degrees with asymptomatic spondylolysis or mild spondylolisthesis (Meyerding grade ≥ I), surgery should focus on the treatment of idiopathic scoliosis (**Fig. 11.5**). However, if the scoliosis is well controlled by conservative treatment while the spondylolisthesis becomes symptomatic (painful) or slippage

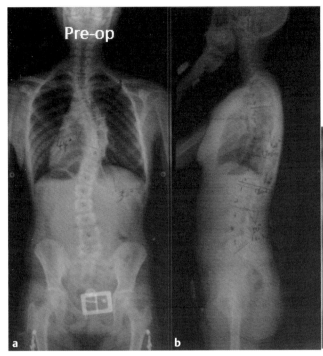

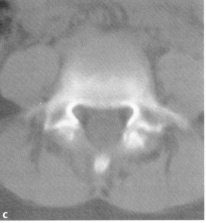

Fig. 11.5 (a–c) Radiographs of a 13-year-old girl with idiopathic thoracic scoliosis (46 degrees) associated with grade I isthmic spondylolisthesis at L5-S1. **(d–g)** The thoracic curve was well corrected and slippage did not progress at 2-year follow-up.

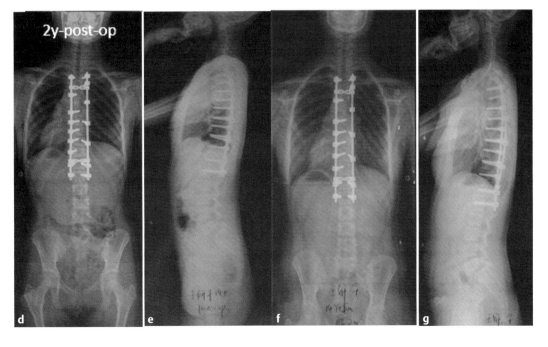

progresses during follow-up, the spondylolisthesis should be treated surgically. If spondylolisthesis is symptomatic, with a Cobb angle of idiopathic scoliosis of more than 45 to 50 degrees, both the scoliosis and spondylolisthe-

sis should be treated with one-stage surgery[6] (**Fig. 11.6**).

As for the olisthetic scoliosis (type II), which is considered to be functional scoliosis, most authors believe it originates from a rotational

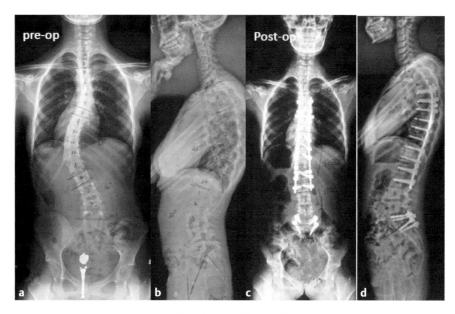

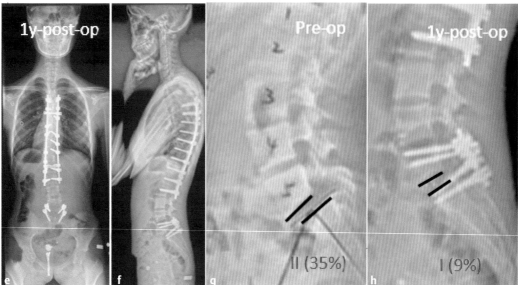

Fig. 11.6 Radiographs of a 14-year-old girl with adolescent isthmic spondylolisthesis associated with idiopathic scoliosis who presented complaining of progressive low back pain and left-sided L5 radiculopathy. The thoracic curve was 50 degrees and grade II slippage was noted. **(a,b,g)** The scoliosis was corrected to 16 degrees, and the spondylolisthesis was treated by posterior instrumentation bilaterally from **(c,d)** L5–S1. **(e,f,h)** The main curve reduced to 14 degrees and the slippage remained grade I at 1-year follow-up.

spondylolytic slip, despite Schlenzka's[15] above-stated doubts. Surgery for reduction and stabilization of the spondylolisthesis is the only required intervention, as scoliosis correction is unnecessary. Earlier studies suggested that the indication for this surgery is grade II or greater spondylolisthesis,[6] regardless of the curve severity or the presence of spondylolisthesis-related symptoms. Posterior surgery by reduction and instrumentation and fusion for spondylolisthesis would be the only required intervention, which can relieve spondylolisthesis-related symptoms as well as achieve a significant improvement of the scoliosis during the follow-up (**Fig. 11.4**). Zhou et al[8] reported a case in which additional surgery for a thoracic curve of 50 degrees was not required after the high-grade spondylolisthesis was well reduced. During the follow-up period, the scoliosis resolved spontaneously (**Fig. 11.7**). However, it remains controversial whether complete decompression or full reduction are necessary. Sailhan et al[16] suggested that a posterior instrumented reduction and fusion of spondylolisthesis without decompression could achieve acceptable radio-graphic and clinical results. However, Zhou et al recommended also performing a posterior decompression because it enabled clear visualization of the nerve roots and helped prevent iatrogenic nerve injury in the process of reduction, and at the same time facilitated performing a diskectomy, a sacral dome osteotomy, and a local nerve decompression if necessary. Some surgeons believe that full slippage reduction is not necessary for these patients. Smith et al[17] reported that partial reduction is an effective technique for the management of high-grade spondylolisthesis. Based on my experience, I prefer to perform a partial reduction and a sacral dome resection for this type of deformity. Interbody cage should be used whenever possible to attain a good sagittal alignment and a satisfactory fusion rate.

Sciatic scoliosis (type III) is also a functional curve, resulting from nerve root compression or stretching, and occurring mainly in association with high-grade spondylolisthesis. This entity, usually manifesting as severe coronal imbalance, shares the same treatment algorithm with the olisthetic scoliosis: posterior

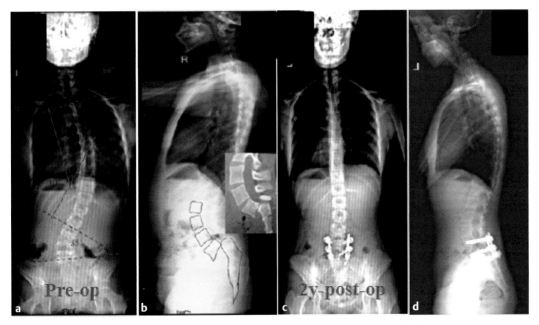

Fig. 11.7 (a,b) The Cobb angle of the main curve is 50 degrees and Meyerding grade IV olisthetic spondylolisthesis is seen at L5–S1. **(c,d)** The scoliosis reached a complete resolution, and the complete correction of L5–S1 spondylolisthesis was well preserved 2 years after surgery. (Courtesy of Yueming Song.)

decompression, instrumentation, reduction, and fusion. Srivastava et al[7] reported that these patients were treated with posterior decompression and transforaminal lumbar interbody fusion (TLIF), demonstrating that this strategy not only can relieve low back pain and L5 radiculopathy, but also can achieve a significant resolution of the scoliosis along with restitution of coronal balance. Although these authors regarded these cases as spondylolisthesis with late-onset idiopathic scoliosis, Schlenzka[15] preferred to describe them as sciatic scoliosis, due to the patients' typical clinical features of a sciatic curve: radicular pain, hamstring tightness,

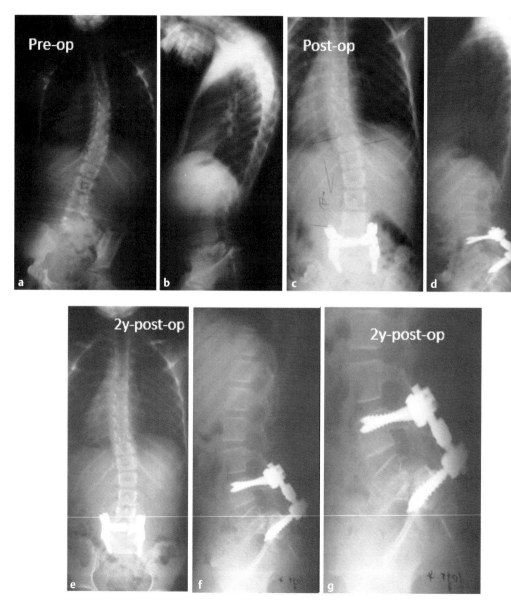

Fig. 11.8 Radiographs of a 10-year-old girl with sciatic scoliosis secondary to dysplastic spondylolisthesis with severe coronal imbalance. **(a,b)** Thoracic curve was 31 degrees and slippage was grade V. **(c,d)** The thoracic curve reduced to 18 degrees after posterior instrumentation from L4 to S1 with partial reduction of spondylolisthesis. **(e–g)** The long curve reduced to 13 degrees and the slippage remained grade II and coronal balance was restored at 2-year follow-up.

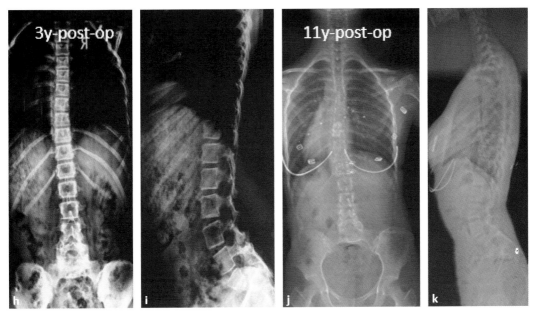

Fig. 11.8 (*continued*) Although the instrumentation was removed 3 year after operation, **(h–k)** spondylolisthesis remains stable without reoccurrence of scoliosis during the next 8 years.

and severe coronal imbalance in adolescents with a high-grade slippage. In my experience, posterior surgery for spondylolisthesis provides more spontaneous correction of sciatic scoliosis (**Fig. 11.8**) than does sciatic scoliosis secondary to lumbar disk herniation.[18]

Chapter Summary

The management of adolescent spondylolisthesis associated with scoliosis remains a great challenge.

The optimal treatment for adolescent scoliosis associated with spondylolisthesis varies based on the type. For idiopathic scoliosis with spondylolisthesis (type I), the two pathologies should be treated separately and the treatment strategy should depend on the curve magnitude of the idiopathic scoliosis and the degree of spondylolisthesis. For types II and III, although the necessity of decompression and perfect reduction remains controversial, surgical treatment for spondylolisthesis not only can relieve the spondylolisthesis-related symptoms, but

also can achieve a significant resolution of the scoliosis along with restoration of coronal balance.

Pearls

◆ There are three types of scoliosis associated with spondylolisthesis: idiopathic scoliosis with spondylolisthesis, olisthetic scoliosis, and sciatic scoliosis.
◆ Adolescent scoliosis associated with spondylolisthesis may progress together with the increasing slippage of the spondylolisthesis during the growth spurts.
◆ The optimal treatment for scoliosis associated with spondylolisthesis varies based on the type. In type I, the two pathologies should be treated separately; in types II and III, the spondylolisthesis should be treated first by posterior decompression, instrumentation, and fusion.

Pitfall

◆ In adolescent scoliosis associated with spondylolisthesis, the curve may evolve together with the upgrading of the spondylolisthesis during growth spurts.

References

Five Must-Read References

1. Cavalier R, Herman MJ, Cheung EV, Pizzutillo PD. Spondylolysis and spondylolisthesis in children and adolescents: I. Diagnosis, natural history, and non-surgical management. J Am Acad Orthop Surg 2006; 14:417–424

2. Seitsalo S, Osterman K, Poussa M. Scoliosis associated with lumbar spondylolisthesis. A clinical survey of 190 young patients. Spine 1988;13:899–904

3. Fisk JR, Moe JH, Winter RB. Scoliosis, spondylolysis, and spondylolisthesis. Their relationship as reviewed in 539 patients. Spine 1978;3:234–245

4. Fredrickson BE, Baker D, McHolick WJ, Yuan HA, Lubicky JP. The natural history of spondylolysis and spondylolisthesis. J Bone Joint Surg Am 1984;66: 699–707

5. Seitsalo S, Osterman K, Hyvärinen H, Tallroth K, Schlenzka D, Poussa M. Progression of spondylolisthesis in children and adolescents. A long-term follow-up of 272 patients. Spine 1991;16:417–421

6. Crostelli M, Mazza O. AIS and spondylolisthesis. Eur Spine J 2013;22(Suppl 2):S172–184

7. Srivastava A, Bayley E, Boszczyk BM. The management of high-grade spondylolisthesis and co-existent late-onset idiopathic scoliosis. Eur Spine J 2016;25: 3027–3031

8. Zhou Z, Song Y, Cai Q, Kong Q. Spontaneous resolution of scoliosis associated with lumbar spondylolisthesis. Spine J 2013;13:e7–e10

9. Crostelli M, Mazza O. Comments about Zou Z, Song Y, Cai Q, Kong Q. Spontaneous resolution of scoliosis associated with lumbar spondylolisthesis. Spine J 2013;13:e7-e10. Spine J 2014;14:1082–1083

10. Périé D, Curnier D. Effect of pathology type and severity on the distribution of MRI signal intensities within the degenerated nucleus pulposus: application to idiopathic scoliosis and spondylolisthesis. BMC Musculoskelet Disord 2010;11:189

11. Koptan WM, El Miligui YH, El Sharkawi MM. Direct repair of spondylolysis presenting after correction of adolescent idiopathic scoliosis. Spine J 2011;11:133–138

12. Libson E, Bloom RA, Shapiro Y. Scoliosis in young men with spondylolysis or spondylolisthesis. A comparative study in symptomatic and asymptomatic subjects. Spine 1984;9:445–447

13. Pneumaticos SG, Esses SI. Scoliosis associated with lumbar spondylolisthesis: a case presentation and review of the literature. Spine J 2003;3:321–324

14. Tojner H. Olisthetic scoliosis. Acta Orthop Scand 1963;33:291–300

15. Schlenzka D. Expert's comment concerning Grand Rounds case entitled "The management of high-grade spondylolisthesis and co-existent late-onset idiopathic scoliosis" (Abhishek Srivastava, Edward Bayley, Bronek M. Boszczyk). Eur Spine J 2016;25: 3032–3033

16. Sailhan F, Gollogly S, Roussouly P. The radiographic results and neurologic complications of instrumented reduction and fusion of high-grade spondylolisthesis without decompression of the neural elements: a retrospective review of 44 patients. Spine 2006;31: 161–169, discussion 170

17. Smith JA, Deviren V, Berven S, Kleinstueck F, Bradford DS. Clinical outcome of trans-sacral interbody fusion after partial reduction for high-grade l5-s1 spondylolisthesis. Spine 2001;26:2227–2234

18. Zhu Z, Zhao Q, Wang B, et al. Scoliotic posture as the initial symptom in adolescents with lumbar disc herniation: its curve pattern and natural history after lumbar discectomy. BMC Musculoskelet Disord 2011; 12:216

Pediatric Spondylolysis and Spondylolisthesis

Michael LaBagnara, Durga R. Sure, Justin S. Smith, and Christopher I. Shaffrey

Introduction

The term *spondylolysis* refers to a defect in the pars interarticularis, which can occur either unilaterally or bilaterally. Spondylolysis is most common in the lumbar spine, with L5 more frequently involved than L4, and other levels involved much less frequently. It may rarely occur at multiple contiguous levels. Approximately 80% of cases involve bilateral pars defects, which can result in the functional separation of the posterior column from the anterior and middle columns. This can result in an anterior translation of the cephalad vertebral body on the caudal level and is termed spondylolisthesis.[1] Spondylolysis is one of the common causes of spondylolisthesis in the pediatric population. These two entities are the most frequent causes of low back pain in pediatric patients. This chapter discusses pediatric spondylolysis and low-grade spondylolisthesis (LGS).

Epidemiology

Spondylolysis and spondylolisthesis are two of the most common identifiable causes of low back pain in children and adolescents. The true incidence of either pathology is difficult to assess, as both are often asymptomatic. The reported incidence of spondylolysis is 4 to 5% by age 6, and increases to 6% by age 18.[1] The male-to-female ratio is 2:1, but females with spondylolysis are more likely to develop spondylolisthesis.[2] The incidence of spondylolysis is highest in adolescent athletes with low back pain, where rates as high 47%[3] to 50%[4] have been reported. Compared with the general pediatric population, a fourfold increase in incidence of spondylolysis has been reported in gymnasts and American football linemen.[5] Spondylolisthesis is more common at L5-S1 in both children and adolescents.[1] Although spondylolysis is more common at L5 than at L4, patients with L4 spondylolysis are more frequently symptomatic.[6]

Pathophysiology

The junction of the relatively mobile lumbar spine and the relatively immobile sacrum results in the L5-S1 joints and L5 pars absorbing more stress than any other level of the spine.[7] With standing posture and weight bearing, the L5-S1 disk resists compression, and shear forces are resisted by the posterior bony-ligamentous complex. The junction of these two anatomic regions is the pars, which is thus exposed to both shear and compressive forces. Incomplete or delayed ossification of the pars, combined with excessive physiological strain can result in a pars stress reaction, which is the precursor to spondylolysis. A pars stress reaction is defined as sclerosis of the pars without a definite radiographic gap. With repetitive mechanical stress the sclerotic bone can fracture, resulting in spondylolysis.[1]

Spondylolysis has not been reported in nonambulatory patients,[8] suggesting that upright posture and ambulation are integral to its development. Spondylolysis is most common in adolescent athletes involved with gymnastics and diving and in adolescent ballet dancers; it is also common in athletes who play contact sports such as American football. Cadaveric biomechanical studies have shown that excessive flexion and extension produce the highest stress on the pars.[7] Of these actions, repetitive hyperextension or the "nutcracker" mechanism is believed to be the most responsible for the development of spondylolysis.[9] More recent studies that evaluated spinopelvic alignment have shown that patients with a large pelvic incidence more frequently have spondylolysis, suggesting that sheer forces also play a major role in the development of spondylolysis.

The development of spondylolisthesis is multifactorial; disk degeneration, ligamentous laxity, genetic predisposition, spina bifida, facet joint incompetency, and spondylolysis can all cause spondylolisthesis, either individually or in combination. Spondylolisthesis may also be iatrogenic. The commonality these factors all share is a functional failure of the posterior bone and ligamentous elements, and this loss of the posterior tension band enables anterior translation of the superior vertebra on the inferior vertebra. In the pediatric population, spondylolysis is the most common cause of spondylolisthesis, attributing to 14 to 21% of cases in previously reported series.[1,10] In patients followed over a 45-year period, Beutler and colleagues[2] observed that those with unilateral spondylolysis typically did not develop spondylolisthesis.

▒ Classification of Spondylolisthesis

There are several classification systems for spondylolisthesis. Both the Wiltse-Newman and the newer Machetti-Bartolozzi systems use etiologic criteria as the basis for classification, whereas the Meyerding, Newman, and DeWald system describes the degree of translation.

The Wiltse-Newman is the oldest and the most commonly used classification of spondylolisthesis (**Table 12.1**). Type I, dysplastic, results from structural abnormalities of the L5-S1 facet joints such as hypoplasia, or malorientation and sacral deficiency. Type II, isthmic, results from defects of the pars interarticularis. Type II is further subcategorized as follows: type IIA, pars lysis; type IIB, pars elongation; and type IIC, acute fracture. Type III results

Table 12.1 Wiltse-Newman Classification

Type	Characteristics
I	Dysplastic
II	Isthmic IIA: pars defect due to fatigue fracture IIB: elongation of pars without disruption secondary to repeated and healed microfractures IIC: pars defect due to acute fracture
III	Degenerative
IV	Traumatic (fracture of posterior elements other than pars)
V	Pathological

Table 12.2 Machetti-Bartolozzi classification

Major Types	Subtypes
Developmental	*High dysplastic*
	With lysis
	With elongation
	Low dysplastic
	With lysis
	With elongation
Acquired	*Traumatic*
	Acute fracture
	Stress fracture
	Postsurgery
	Direct surgery
	Indirect surgery
	Pathological
	Local pathology
	Systemic pathology
	Degenerative
	Primary
	Secondary

Table 12.3 Meyerding Classification

Grade	Extent of Vertebral Slippage
I	< 25%
II	25–49%
III	50–74%
IV	≥ 75%
V	Spondyloptosis

from degenerative disease. Type IV results from traumatic fracture of the posterior elements other than the pars. Type V is due to pathological destruction of the posterior elements.

Machetti and Bartolozzi subsequently proposed a classification that differentiates developmental and acquired types (**Table 12.2**).[11] In this classification, Wiltse I and II are grouped together as developmental. Degenerative, pathological, and traumatic causes are grouped into an acquired category.

Lastly, the Meyerding classification is a radiographic classification (**Table 12.3**).[11]

The importance of spinopelvic parameters and global sagittal alignment, specifically with respect to treatment decisions in spondylolisthesis, has been demonstrated in the literature.[9,11–13] The previously discussed classification systems do not include these measurements of spinopelvic alignment or balance.

In 2006, Mac-Thiong and colleagues[11] proposed a new classification system based on the degree of slippage, the degree of dysplasia, and the sagittal spinopelvic balance. They described nine types and proposed tentative treatment guidelines based on the degree of severity.

More recently, the Spinal Deformity Study Group (SDSG) proposed a simplified classification system for L5-S1 spondylolisthesis (**Table 12.4**).[12] It is based on the degree of listhesis, the pelvis type, and the spinopelvic balance. Based on these three parameters, the SDSG created six subtypes. The degree of slippage is either low grade (< 50%) or high grade (≥ 50%). The spinopelvic measurements of pelvic incidence (PI), pelvic tilt (PT), sacral slope (SS), and C7 plumb line (C7PL) are used to classify the pelvis as balanced, retroverted with a balanced spine, or retroverted with an unbalanced spine. Low-grade spondylolistheses is one of three types: type I, low PI (< 45 degrees); type II, normal PI (45 to 60 degrees); and type III, high PI (> 60 degrees).

Higher grade slips similarly fit into three types: type IV, balanced pelvis; type V, retroverted pelvis with a balanced spine; and type VI, retroverted pelvis with an unbalanced spine. The spine is considered "balanced" if the C7PL falls on or behind the femoral heads, and unbalanced if it falls anterior to the femoral heads.

Utilization of this classification system for higher grade spondylolisthesis has been shown to improve surgical decision making.[12]

Table 12.4 Spinal Deformity Study Group (SDSG) Classification

Low grade	Type I: PI < 45 degrees
	Type II: PI = 45 to 60 degrees
	Type III: PI > 60 degrees
High grade	Type IV: balanced pelvis
	Type V: retroverted pelvis and balanced spine
	Type VI: retroverted pelvis and unbalanced spine

Abbreviation: PI, pelvic incidence.

Clinical Presentation

Spondylolysis and low-grade spondylolisthesis are often asymptomatic. Symptomatic patients typically present with focal back pain that is exacerbated by activity, particularly activities that involve hyperextension of the lumbar spine. Radicular symptoms may or may not be present.

Diagnostic Imaging

Standing anteroposterior (AP) and lateral radiographs of the lumbar spine are valuable diagnostic tools, as they enable assessment of both spondylolysis and spondylolisthesis at the same time. When combined with oblique views, a unilateral stress reaction or unilateral defect may be visualized; it classically resembles the broken neck of a Scottie dog.

Assessment of global spinal alignment and spinopelvic parameters is strongly recommended once spondylolisthesis has been diagnosed. This can be accomplished with either standing 36-inch AP and lateral radiographs or with any of the ALARA (As Low As Reasonably Achievable) imaging systems. The latter modalities are preferable as they employ significantly lower radiation dosages, provide true-to-size images that aid in surgical planning, and facilitate assessment of the entire spine. Other imaging studies, including computed tomography (CT) and magnetic resonance imaging (MRI), are generally acquired with the patient in the supine position, and although they all provide superior visualization of the bony, ligamentous, and nervous system anatomy, the degree of olisthesis may be underestimated or completely missed. Supine or extension radiographs are recommended, if spondylolisthesis is present, to assess the degree of mobility.

Computed tomography imaging provides superior visualization of the bony anatomy and may also have prognostic significance. Early spondylolytic lesions without sclerosis or significant displacement are easily visualized on sagittal reconstructions.[14] Early spondylolysis without sclerotic lesion findings are more likely to heal with nonoperative therapy including bracing, and are often not visualized on plain radiographs. MRI without contrast enables visualization of the disks, ligaments, joint capsules, and neural elements. MRI should be considered for patients with neurologic symptoms. A T2 hyperintensity within the pars or pedicle may be visualized in early lesions, and when present, has prognostic value. Single photon emission computed tomography (SPECT) imaging can be added to evaluate the metabolic activity within the pars, and it is more sensitive for identifying "occult" fractures that the other modalities may fail to detect. Metabolically active or "hot" lesions are thought to be those that are early in their course, and they tend to respond better to brace and nonoperative management when compared with "cold" lesions that are thought to be more longstanding.[14]

Treatment

Treatment of spondylolysis and spondylolisthesis is based on skeletal age/maturity, the risk of progressive deformity, the presence and severity of symptoms, and the degree of olisthesis, if present.

Nonoperative Treatment

Asymptomatic patients should be managed with observation only, without activity modification. Symptomatic pediatric spondylolysis can often be effectively treated nonoperatively with a combination of activity modification and physiotherapy, with or without an external orthosis. The goal of these measures is to reduce the extension of the lumbar spine, with emphasis on core strengthening and improvement of range of motion of the hip. The combination of activity modification, physiotherapy, with or without an external thoracolumbar orthosis for 3 to 6 months has been shown to be effective for most unilateral and approximately half of bilateral spondylolytic lesions, if they are identified early.[15] There is presently no consensus on the use of an orthosis.

Similarly, the above measures are effective for treating low back pain in children with symptomatic grade I spondylolisthesis. If spondylolisthesis is identified before skeletal maturity, clinical and radiographic evaluation every 6 to 12 months is recommended to evaluate progression. This is especially important for children with dysplastic spondylolisthesis and spina bifida, conditions that are more likely to progress from low to high grade. The goal of nonoperative management for LGS is symptomatic improvement and return to function. Surgical therapy should be considered for patients with persistent or worsening symptoms after 6 months of appropriate conservative therapy or evidence of significant slippage progression.

Surgical Treatment

Spondylolysis

Spondylolytic defects can be repaired directly or treated with fusion to the subjacent vertebra with surgical therapy. Prior to a surgeon recommending direct repair, the patient should be referred for percutaneous injection of local anesthetic, with or without corticosteroid, directly into the defect. Symptomatic improvement following injection is a strong prognostic indicator of success with direct repair.[3] When possible, direct repair is preferred over segmental instrumentation and fusion as it maintains segmental mobility.[16] Thus, it should be

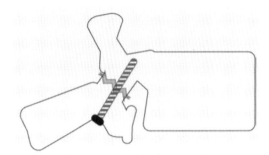

Fig. 12.1 Single lag screw (Buck technique).

considered for both unilateral and bilateral defects that remain symptomatic after appropriate conservative management.

Direct repair is contraindicated in the presence of significant disk degeneration, facet disease, segmental instability, spina bifida, or dysplastic bony changes. Additionally, direct repair of spondylolysis at L5 has been suggested to have suboptimal results when compared with fusion procedures, which may be related to the pars elongation and the increased dynamic forces most commonly seen at this level.[17] Pseudarthrosis following direct repair is more common in patients over 20 years of age, and in treating defects larger than 2 mm.[18]

Direct repair involves debridement of the pars defect, autologous iliac crest bone grafting, and distal fragment stabilization. There are several possible constructs for stabilizing the distal fragment, including tension band wiring, a single lag screw (Buck technique, **Fig. 12.1**), screw-hook fixation (Morscher, **Fig. 12.2**), cerclage wire fixation to the spinous process below (Scott), pedicle screw cable fixation (Songer, **Fig. 12.3**), pedicle screw hook fixation

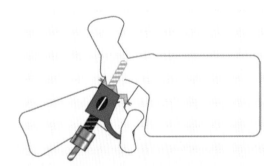

Fig. 12.2 Screw-hook fixation (Morscher).

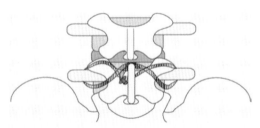

Fig. 12.3 Pedicle screw cable fixation (Songer).

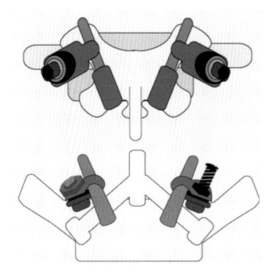

Fig. 12.4 Pedicle screw hook fixation.

(**Fig. 12.4**), and bilateral pedicle screw and U-shaped rod fixation to the spinous process below (**Fig. 12.5**).[14] Success or failure of the procedure is less dependent on the type of construct than on the construct's ability to apply compression across the graft. The published literature regarding the success of these techniques is limited to small cohort studies of mostly less than 100 patients. Although there is presently no consensus on the superiority of any one construct, a recent meta-analysis reported good to excellent outcomes following direct repair in excess of 60% and as high as 90%.[14]

Ideal candidates for direct repair include athletes under 20 years of age who have failed appropriate nonoperative management and who wish to return to competing in their sport. Direct repair enables aggressive physical therapy and strengthening after the initial postoperative pain has subsided. Successful direct repair not only provides the restoration of "normal" anatomy (without loss of motion segments), but also is reported to have the best chance of the patient returning to sports.[14] There is presently no consensus on how long after surgery return to play is appropriate. Most series report between 5 and 7 months for noncontact sports and up to 12 months for contact sports, although this is patient and surgeon dependent. Posterolateral fusion with pedicle screw fixation should be considered for failed direct repair (pseudarthrosis) and in patients over 20 years of age.

Low-Grade Spondylolisthesis

As previously stated, spondylolysis with concomitant spondylolisthesis is a contraindication to direct repair of the pars. In this setting, appropriate nonoperative management should be pursued before invasive treatment is considered.

The two primary surgical options for treatment of pediatric LGS are instrumented fusion and noninstrumented fusion. Noninstrumented fusion and an external orthosis were previously the mainstay for treatment, although advances in instrumentation over the preceding decades have changed this viewpoint for the majority of surgeons. Bilateral pedicle screw fixation and posterolateral fusion, with or without decompression and with or without interbody fusion, have largely replaced noninstrumented fusion.

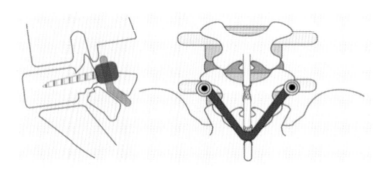

Fig. 12.5 Bilateral pedicle screw and U-shaped rod fixation to the spinous process below.

Interbody fusion and direct decompression of neural elements are both associated with higher complication rates than posterolateral fusion alone. These complications are mainly dural tear/cerebrospinal fluid (CSF) leak and a new neurologic deficit. Interbody fusion is associated with higher fusion rates, improved reduction of olisthesis, and indirect decompression of neural elements. There is presently no consensus on the use of interbody fusion or direct decompression for treatment of LGS in the pediatric population, as there are no studies on comparative effectiveness, and many series have few patients requiring surgery, especially when compared with high-grade spondylolisthesis (HGS).[19,20]

▩ Case Example

A 17-year-old male lacrosse and football player initially presented to the senior author with low back pain exacerbated by activity. Preoperative AP and flexion and extension radiographs (**Figs. 12.6** and **12.7**) were obtained, as

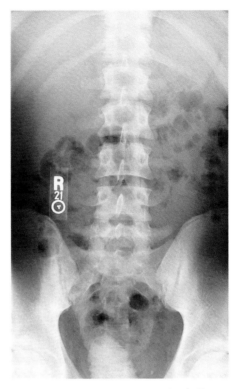

Fig. 12.6 Preoperative anteroposterior (AP) radiograph.

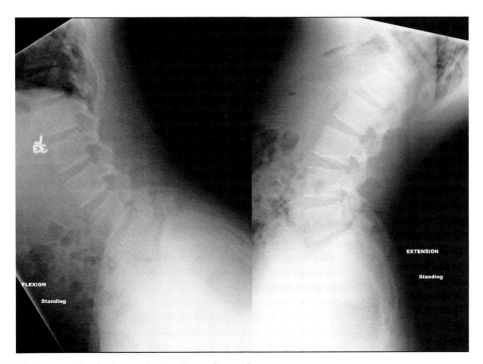

Fig. 12.7 Preoperative flexion and extension radiograph.

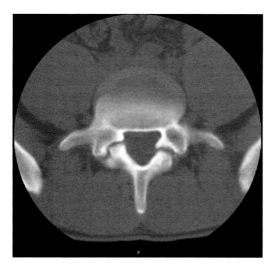

Fig. 12.8 Axial preoperative computed tomography (CT).

were axial and sagittal CT scans through the affected level (**Figs. 12.8** and **12.9**). Sagittal T2 MRI demonstrated a lack of significant degeneration of the L5-S1 disk (**Fig. 12.10**).

The patient underwent direct repair with a hook-screw construct. Postoperative AP and bilateral oblique radiographs were obtained (**Figs. 12.11** and **12.12**). An axial CT scan obtained 4 months after surgery demonstrated fusion across the pars. The patient subsequently returned to competing in lacrosse and football at the collegiate level.

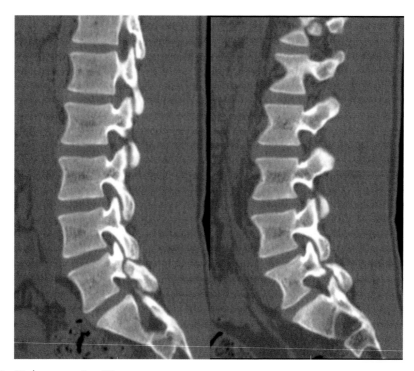

Fig. 12.9 Sagittal preoperative CT.

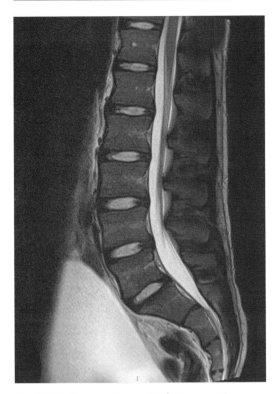

Fig. 12.10 Preoperative sagittal T2 magnetic resonance imaging (MRI).

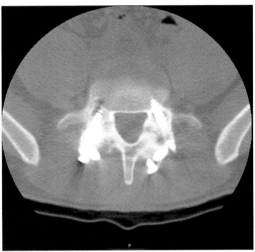

Fig. 12.11 Postoperative axial CT scan.

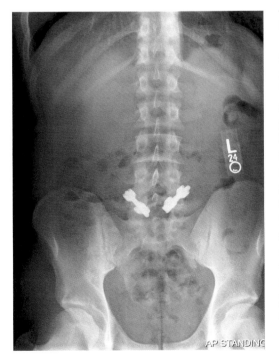

Fig. 12.12 Post AP radiograph.

▥ Chapter Summary

Spondylolysis and LGS are relatively uncommon entities within the pediatric population. They are especially common in adolescent athletes, and classically present with low back pain that is exacerbated by activity, particularly hyperextension of the lumbar spine. Early spondylolysis and LGS respond well to nonoperative measures of activity modification and physiotherapy, with or without an external orthosis. Direct surgical repair of symptomatic spondylolytic defects should be considered for competitive athletes who have failed conservative management, as direct repair provides the highest chance for return to play. In the presence of olisthesis or symptomatic subjacent disk degeneration, fusion with or without interbody arthrodesis is appropriate.

- ◆ Direct repair of spondylolysis is contraindicated in the presence of olisthesis, significant facet disease, disk degeneration, segmental instability, spina bifida, or bony dysplasia.
- ◆ Direct repair of spondylolysis entails higher rates of pseudarthrosis for patients over 20 years of age and defects greater than 2 mm.
- ◆ When LGS is identified before skeletal maturity, patients should be followed clinically and radiographically every 6 to 12 months until skeletal maturity to search for the presence of slip progression.

- ◆ Pay careful attention to advanced imaging; the presence of dysplastic bony changes, disk degeneration, and facet disease are important factors in surgical decision making.
- ◆ Do not fail to obtain upright radiographs, including dynamic imaging.

References

Five Must-Read References

1. Cavalier R, Herman MJ, Cheung EV, Pizzutillo PD. Spondylolysis and spondylolisthesis in children and adolescents: I. Diagnosis, natural history, and nonsurgical management. J Am Acad Orthop Surg 2006; 14:417–424
2. Beutler WJ, Fredrickson BE, Murtland A, Sweeney CA, Grant WD, Baker D. The natural history of spondylolysis and spondylolisthesis: 45-year follow-up evaluation. Spine 2003;28:1027–1035, discussion 1035
3. Micheli LJ, Wood R. Back pain in young athletes. Significant differences from adults in causes and patterns. Arch Pediatr Adolesc Med 1995;149:15–18
4. Sassmannshausen G, Smith BG. Back pain in the young athlete. Clin Sports Med 2002;21:121–132
5. Jackson DW, Wiltse LL, Cirincoine RJ. Spondylolysis in the female gymnast. Clin Orthop Relat Res 1976; 117:68–73
6. Saraste H. Long-term clinical and radiological follow-up of spondylolysis and spondylolisthesis. J Pediatr Orthop 1987;7:631–638
7. Dietrich M, Kurowski P. The importance of mechanical factors in the etiology of spondylolysis. A model analysis of loads and stresses in human lumbar spine. Spine 1985;10:532–542
8. Rosenberg NJ, Bargar WL, Friedman B. The incidence of spondylolysis and spondylolisthesis in nonambulatory patients. Spine 1981;6:35–38
9. Labelle H, Roussouly P, Berthonnaud E, et al. Spondylolisthesis, pelvic incidence, and spinopelvic balance: a correlation study. Spine 2004;29:2049–2054
10. Boxall D, Bradford DS, Winter RB, Moe JH. Management of severe spondylolisthesis in children and adolescents. J Bone Joint Surg Am 1979;61:479–495
11. Mac-Thiong JM, Labelle H. A proposal for a surgical classification of pediatric lumbosacral spondylolisthesis based on current literature. Eur Spine J 2006;15: 1425–1435
12. Labelle H, Mac-Thiong JM, Roussouly P. Spino-pelvic sagittal balance of spondylolisthesis: a review and classification. Eur Spine J 2011;20(Suppl 5):641–646
13. Hresko MT, Labelle H, Roussouly P, Berthonnaud E. Classification of high-grade spondylolistheses based on pelvic version and spine balance: possible rationale for reduction. Spine 2007;32:2208–2213
14. Drazin D, Shirzadi A, Jeswani S. Direct surgical repair of spondylolysis in athletes: Indications, techniques, and outcomes. Neurosurg Focus 2011;31:E9
15. Morita T, Ikata T, Katoh S, Miyake R. Lumbar spondylolysis in children and adolescents. J Bone Joint Surg Br 1995;77B:620–625
16. Snyder LA, Shufflebarger H, O'Brien MF, Thind H, Theodore N, Kakarla UK. Spondylolysis outcomes in adolescents after direct screw repair of the pars interarticularis. J Neurosurg Spine 2014;21:329–333
17. Tsirikos AI, Garrido EG. Spondylolysis and spondylolisthesis in children and adolescents. J Bone Joint Surg Br 2010;92:751–759
18. Ivanic GM, Pink TP, Achatz W, Ward JC, Homann NC, May M. Direct stabilization of lumbar spondylolysis with a hook screw: mean 11-year follow-up period for 113 patients. Spine 2003;28:255–259
19. Kasliwal MK, Smith JS, Shaffrey CI, et al. Short-term complications associated with surgery for high-grade spondylolisthesis in adults and pediatric patients: a report from the scoliosis research society morbidity and mortality database. Neurosurgery 2012;71:109–116
20. Fu KM, Smith JS, Polly DW Jr, et al. Morbidity and mortality in the surgical treatment of six hundred five pediatric patients with isthmic or dysplastic spondylolisthesis. Spine 2011;36:308–312

13

Dysplastic High-Grade Spondylolisthesis

Yazeed M. Gussous and Sigurd H. Berven

Introduction

Spondylolysis and spondylolisthesis are a common cause of low back pain in the adolescent. Spondylolisthesis in the child presents with deformity of the lumbopelvic segment, malalignment of global sagittal balance, and clinical signs and symptoms in a range of severity. The term *dysplastic high-grade spondylolisthesis* describes both the severity and the etiology of the deformity. High-grade olisthesis encompasses a deformity of L5 that has slipped forward on S1 by more than 50%. Dysplasia describes an etiology that is related to malformation of the L5-S1 segment of the spine, which may include a high pelvic incidence (PI) with incomplete formation of the posterior elements of L5-S1 including the facet joints. Dysplastic high-grade spondylolisthesis at L5-S1 accounts for 15% of spondylolisthesis presenting before adulthood.[1–3] It affects children's health-related quality of life (HRQOL), and presents the risk of deformity progression and development of neural symptoms and dysfunction.

The evaluation and management of high-grade dysplastic spondylolisthesis is controversial, especially regarding the goal of reducing the high-grade deformity and the role for interbody support. This chapter reviews the classification and etiology of spondylolisthesis in the child, and discusses the indications for, and details of, specific surgical techniques for the management of dysplastic high-grade spondylolisthesis in children.

Classification Systems

Numerous classification systems have been proposed in the literature for the etiology and pathology of spondylolisthesis. More recent classifications helped us develop an understanding of the concepts of sacropelvic and spinopelvic balance and their role in guiding decision making in surgical planning.

Meyerding[4] Classification

Henry Meyerding of the Mayo Clinic devised in 1938 a simple classification system based on the percentage of slippage of the vertebra relative to each other.[5] Grade 1 entails a slippage of 25%, grade 2 a slippage of 50%, grade 3 a slippage of 75%, grade 4 a slippage up to 100%, and grade 5 a slippage of more than 100% or spondyloptosis. Low-grade olisthesis generally refers to slippage of grade 2 or less and high grade spondylolisthesis refers to slippage of grade 3 or more. The advantages of this classification system are that it is easy to remember and it is highly reproducible, with good inter- and intraobserver reproducibility. However, it does not include important descriptive variables of the slippage, such as the angular kyphotic deformation at the lumbosacral junction.

Wiltse and MacNab Classification

In 1976, Wiltse et al[2] described an etiology-based classification system for spondylolisthesis that includes five types of spondylolisthesis and three subtypes of the type II (**Table 13.1**). The discussion in this chapter is mainly concerned with the type I, dysplastic spondylolisthesis.

Marchetti and Bartolozzi[7] Classification

This is an etiology-based system proposed in 1982 that classifies spondylolisthesis into two broad categories: acquired and developmental. The two categories are further subdivided (**Table 13.2**). This chapter is mainly focused on the high dysplastic subtype in the developmental category.

Mac-Thiong Classification

Mac-Thiong et al[8] and Labelle proposed a classification system that incorporated the concept of sagittal spinopelvic balance and sacropelvic balance to help guide surgical planning. This is a very important concept for our discussion of the treatment of dysplastic high-grade spondylolisthesis as it has therapeutic implications for patients.

The concept of sacropelvic balance culminated from the study of various patterns of high or low PI and high or low sacral slope (SS), which affect the biomechanics at the lumbosacral junction in different ways. Hresko used cluster analysis to define two subsets of subjects with high-grade spondylolisthesis: patients with a balanced sacropelvic relationship had a high SS and a low pelvic tilt (PT), whereas patients with a low SS and a high PT had a retroverted pelvic and vertical sacrum along with lumbosacral kyphosis and sacropelvic imbalance.

The mechanism of compensation for various degrees of lumbosacral imbalance depends on the severity of the imbalance. As imbalance develops, an increase in lumbar lordosis maintains the center of gravity over the hips. However, as the maximal lordosis is attained, the pelvis must be retroverted to keep the center of gravity over the hips. The relationship PI = SS + PT dictates that with the decrease in SS, the PT must increase to maintain balance. According to Mac-Thiong and Labelle, once the anatomic limit of these mechanisms is reached, sagittal spinal imbalance results, forcing the subject to lean forward.

The significance of the Mac-Thiong classification is that it suggests treatment options based on grade. This treatment algorithm, however, needs to be corroborated with more evidence to support it. The low-grade group is further divided into low PI/low SS (nutcracker subtype) or high PI/low SS (shear subtype). In general, those with low-grade spondylolisthesis according to the Mac-Thiong classification

Table 13.1 Wiltse Classification[6]

Type	Description
I	Dysplastic
II-A	Isthmic: pars fatigue
II-B	Isthmic: pars elongation due to multiple healed stress fractures
II-C	Isthmic: pars acute fracture
III	Degenerative: facet instability without pars fracture
IV	Traumatic: acute posterior arch fracture other than pars fatigue fracture
V	Neoplastic: pathologic destruction of the pars leading to deformity

Table 13.2 Marchetti and Bartolozzi Classification

Type	Subtype
Developmental	High dysplastic
	Low dysplastic
Acquired	Traumatic
	Degenerative
	Pathological (local or systemic)
	Postsurgical (direct or indirect)

scheme are proposed to be best served by an in situ posterolateral fusion, which has a favorable fusion rate regardless of instrumentation.

The high-grade subtype is further divided into balanced pelvis or imbalanced pelvis, as described above. Patients with imbalanced pelvis are further subdivided into those with an imbalanced spine sagittally and those with a balanced spine sagittally. Although intraobserver reliability was high for this classification system, the interobserver reliability was only moderate because of the difficulty in classifying the degree of the dysplasia.

Spinal Deformity Study Group Classification

The classification proposed by the Spinal Deformity Study Group (SDSG) is a modification of the Mac-Thiong Classification.[9,10] The current version of this system has been simplified when compared with the previous version. First, determine whether the slippage is low grade (Meyerding 1 or 2) or high grade (Meyerding 3 or 4). Next, measure the sacropelvic parameters of SS and PT, and calculate PI. For low-grade spondylolisthesis, two subgroups are divided at a PI value of 60 degrees. For high-grade spondylolisthesis, the Hresko et al method is applied. Patients are assigned to these categories based on the threshold line defined in the cluster analysis. Above the line, the patient is classified as having a balanced pelvis (high SS/low PT); below the line, the patient is classified as having an un balanced pelvis (low SS/high PT). The global spinopelvic balance is also easily determined. If the C7 plumb line falls over or posterior to the femoral head, the spine is balanced. However, if it lies anterior to the femoral heads, the spine is unbalanced. Usually if the sacropelvis is balanced, the patient displays global spinal balance regardless of the grade. However, this may not be the case in patients with high-grade spondylolisthesis with an unbalanced pelvis. A reliability study was performed on this system as well. Using a computer-assisted method of identifying anatomic landmarks, the study was able to demonstrate high reliability in both inter- and intraobserver reliability (**Fig. 13.1**).

Treatment

The majority of patients with spondylolisthesis have lower grade degenerative or isthmic disease that can be treated conservatively. Surgery is appropriate for patients who have failed conservative measures and have a persistent neurologic deficit, intractable pain, instability, or positive sagittal balance with higher grade

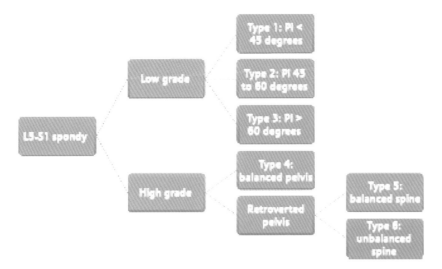

Fig. 13.1 Spinal Deformity Study Group Classification system for L5-S1 spondylolisthesis.

disease. The focus of this discussion in on the treatment of high-grade spondylolisthesis and on surgical techniques for managing dysplastic high-grade spondylolisthesis. The decision to treat high-grade spondylolisthesis with surgery is an area of controversy, and multiple techniques for reduction and fixation have been described.

Patients with high-grade slippage are usually symptomatic, with an imbalanced sacropelvic or spinopelvic relationship; surgical management is generally indicated. The primary goals of treatment in these patients are to relieve the patient's pain and neurologic deficit and to restore the alignment when indicated. Maximizing the fusion area by including anterior fusion or with transsacral fixation is typically necessary. Unbalanced deformities may necessitate reduction of the sagittal malalignment based on the proposed SDSG classification algorithm above, with the suggestion that reduction may be indicated for type 5 and type 6 deformities. In addition, inclusion of full-length lateral 36-inch scoliosis radiographs are imperative to further classify overall sagittal balance.[11,12]

Significant controversy exists regarding the necessity of reducing the slippage, the timing of surgery, and the most effective means of achieving reduction. Although low-grade spondylolistheses treated with in situ fusion have shown relatively good outcomes, high-grade slippages with pelvic imbalance or spinal imbalance treated without reduction are thought to be prone to high rates of nonunion or slippage progression and patient dissatisfaction.

Advocates of in situ fusion report a high rate of back pain relief and a low risk of iatrogenic neurologic deficit. On the other hand, advocates of reduction report a higher fusion rate due to the increased surface area of bone, and improved sagittal balance. Poussa et al[13] found that the in situ fusion group had a 27% rate of pseudarthrosis. Prior studies have shown that patients who undergo reduction have satisfaction scores and outcomes similar to those of patients who undergo in situ fixation. Poussa et al also found that the in situ fusion patients did better in terms of their Oswestry Disability Index (ODI) score and had less adjacent disk degeneration and muscle atrophy as seen on magnetic resonance imaging (MRI); thus, Poussa

et al concluded that in situ fusion is a safer procedure with good long-term outcomes.

Ruf et al[14] found improved radiographic parameters after reduction and fusion, and minimal risk of permanent nerve root damage. A recent systematic review of eight studies also found that reduction improved the overall spine biomechanics and was not associated with a greater risk of neurologic deficits when compared with in situ fixation.

Various methods of reduction and fusion of spondylolisthesis have been described in the literature. Some are of historical significance and are no longer practiced commonly. Some of the historical techniques included halo-femoral traction with pelvic suspension, anterior-posterior in situ fusion and placement of a pantaloons spica cast in hyperextension, use of halo skeletal traction in a staged manner, and use of Magerl's external fixator for reduction. With advancement of surgical techniques and more powerful instrumentation, these historical techniques are no longer utilized.

Reduction of slippage includes reduction of the lumbosacral kyphosis at L5-S1 and reduction of the translation of the L5-S1 vertebrae. The highest yield reduction would be L5-S1 kyphosis in terms of restoring sagittal balance, whereas reduction of the translation helps to further improve the sagittal profile, but also increases the interbody contact area between L5 and S1, improving the fusion potential.

After reduction, fusion can be performed as interbody fusion or through a transsacral fibula graft spanning the L5 segment.

Additional points of fixation up to L4 and down to the pelvis may be needed.

▨ Preoperative Planning

A full history should be taken and a physical examination should be performed. Full-length standing radiographs should be obtained. Determining the patient's neurologic status, adjacent segment degeneration, Meyerding grade, Labelle type, and the status of the sacropelvic and spinopelvic balance will aid in the treatment decision making and preoperative surgical planning.

⫸ Imaging

Measurement of the global sagittal balance and local parameters is essential, including PI, PT, SS, lumbar lordosis, and slip angle. Boxall and Bradford's group[15] demonstrated the importance of the slip angle as a measurement of the percentage of slippage and in predicting progression of the slippage in patients treated with in situ fusion; the slip angle measures the kyphotic relationship of the fifth lumbar to the first sacral vertebra (**Fig. 13.2**).

L5 pedicles are often deficient and may necessitate further temporary or permanent fixation points adjacent to it. The presence of a sacral dome may impede the reduction maneuver and should be taken into consideration to incorporate resection of the sacral dome (so-called sacral dome osteotomy) as part of the procedure.

The partial reduction of L5 on S1 limits the surface area for interbody fusion, and results in residual high shear forces between L5 and S1, which may compromise osseous healing between L5 and S1.

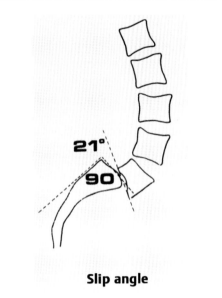

Slip angle

Fig. 13.2 The slip angle measurement. The angle between the lower end plate of L5 and the perpendicular line to the S1 tangent is shown. The percentage of slippage is also depicted (Meyerding grade). (Modified from Boxall D, Bradford DS, Winter RB, Moe JH. Management of severe spondylolisthesis in children and adolescents. J Bone Joint Surg Am 1979;61:479–495.)

⫸ In Situ Fusion with Fibular Allograft

Posterior Based

Bohlman and Cook[16] described the placement of a fibular graft through a posterior transsacral approach from the S1 body across the disk space into the L5 body. This technique obviates the need for an anterior approach, but it entails manipulation of the thecal sac. It is utilized when in situ fusion is intended. A guidewire is advanced through the body of S1, across the L5-S1 disk space, and up to the anterior cortex of L5. Over-reaming of the guidewire can be performed under fluoroscopic guidance with an anterior cruciate ligament (ACL) reamer, beginning at 6 mm and increasing incrementally up to 10 to 12 mm. The donor fibula can be impacted under fluoroscopic guidance. Most surgeons today adopt a modified version of this technique that supplements it with posterior pedicle screw fixation to stabilize the trans-

sacral fusion. The technique may also be used to stabilize the L5-S1 segment after a partial reduction (**Fig. 13.3**). The transsacral fixation with s fibula or structural graft and screws results in rigid fixation between L5 and S1.

Outcomes of partial reduction and transosseous fixation were reported in several retrospective studies. Smith et al[17] reported their technique and experience with a modified Bohlman technique for partial reduction of L5 on S1 and transosseous fixation including transosseous screws and fibula. Improvement in the lumbosacral slip angle by over 20 degrees was seen on radiographs, and clinical outcomes suggested high rates of patient satisfaction.

Hart et al[18] reported outcomes at 5-year follow-up in patients treated with the modified Bohlman technique using partial reduction and transosseous fixation. The slip angle averaged 71 degrees preoperatively, was corrected to an average of 31 degrees by reduction, and averaged 28 degrees at follow-up. The averagepreoperative percentage of slippage (98%) did not change substantially. Radicular pain

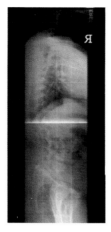
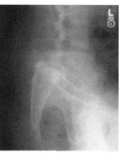
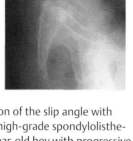
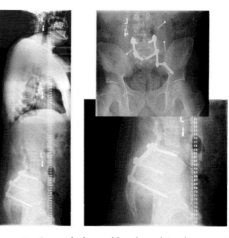

a

b

Fig. 13.3 Partial reduction of the slip angle with transosseous fixation of high-grade spondylolisthesis. The patient is a 17-year-old boy with progressive low back pain, bilateral L5 weakness, and limited standing and walking tolerance. **(a)** Preoperative posteroanterior (PA) and lateral radiographs demonstrating unbalanced lumbopelvic alignment, with balance global spine alignment (type 5). **(b)** Postoperatively, a partial reduction with transosseous fixation results in significant improvement of lumbopelvic alignment and stabilization of the dysplastic olisthesis.

improved in all 12 patients who reported the complaint preoperatively. Ten patients had postoperative neurologic deficits that completely resolved in all but one at follow-up. The authors also reported pseudarthrosis in 21% (four patients).

The modified Bohlman technique was reported by multiple surgeons to show high fusion rates (14 of 16 [88]%). Rates of L5 motor deficit were low in comparison with techniques involving reduction of the anterolisthesis.[18]

Anterior and Posterior

Bradford and Lovett[19] and Bradford and Boachie-Adjei[20] recommended the combined anterior and posterior approaches with complete posterior decompression when the slippage exceeds 75% so as to decrease the risk of pseudarthrosis. To avoid nonunion, interbody fusion through either anterior or posterior approaches provides additional surface for fusion as well as a biomechanical advantage against tensile forces on the posterior fusion. Furthermore, interbody fusion enables wider posterior decompression of neural elements with less concern about nonunion. Also, it facilitates correction of the sagittal alignment and reduction of the deformity.

Gaines[21] popularized a two-stage technique involving excision of the L5 vertebral body along with the L4–L5 and the L5-S1 disks through an anterior approach followed by a posterior approach to excise the loose posterior elements, the articular processes, and the pedicles of L5 with neural decompression and reduction of L4 onto S1 to achieve correction of deformity. This reduction is maintained by posterolateral fusion with transpedicular instrumentation from L4 to S1. This technique is typically reserved for patients with spondyloptosis or grade IV or V spondylolisthesis. Iatrogenic neurologic injury has been reported in up to one third of patients.[22]

All-Posterior Approach

Positioning and Approach

The all-posterior approach is the most often utilized technique for most high-grade slippages. This subsection describes the interbody technique for the all-posterior approach after reduction (**Fig. 13.4**). Another possible technique is to perform the transsacral fusion after

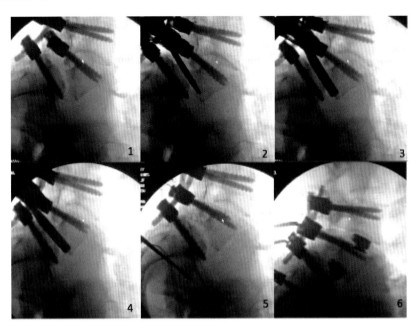

Fig. 13.4 (1–6) This demonstrates the intraoperative radiographs of the steps for posterior-based reduction of L5. (1) Segmental fixation at L4, L5 and S1. (2) Osteotomy to remove dome of the sacrum. (3) Insertion of paddle distractor. (4) Use of paddle distractor to lever L5 into lordotic position. (5) Reduction of L5 onto rod. (6) Placement of interbody cages.

the reduction; this latter modification was first described by Bradford et al.[20]

The patient is placed in a prone position on a modified Jackson table early in the procedure. Pelvic retroversion is maximized by the placement of the hip pads higher and using a sling for positioning the lower extremities; these steps may assist in the decompression of the posterior elements and in exposing the L5-S1 disk for the reduction and fixation correction.

The open procedure utilizes a standard midline exposure. Special care is taken with any dysplastic changes or spina bifida occulta so as to avoid inadvertent dural tears.

Prior to reduction, decompression of the L5 nerve roots should be completed. Subsequent preparation of the involved disk space (resecting the posterior annulus) and removal of the dome of the sacrum is advisable to facilitate later reduction. Posterior fixation may extend from L4 or L5 to the sacrum and pelvis. Iliac fixation is important to reduce stress on the S1 screws. A stiff rod is placed in the S1 with ilium screws and with dorsal displacement of the rod

above L5. This creates a stable post to which the slipped L5 vertebra can be reduced with reduction screws.

An instrument in the disk space such as a Cobb elevator or disk shaver or paddle is useful to cantilever the displaced L5 vertebra posteriorly and into alignment with the sacrum; this reduction maneuver can be performed unilaterally. Additional proximal fixation with L4 screws may be used as a means to reduce the stress on the L5 screws to obtain the reduction of L5. This may be temporary or definitive (and included in the final fusion construct). **Fig. 13.5** demonstrates a posterior-based reduction of dysplastic spondylolisthesis in a 12-year-old girl with high-grade dysplastic spondylolisthesis.

L5 Neurologic Deficit and Reduction

The tension on the L5 nerve root is directly proportional to the percentage of reduction, with the majority of tension (71%) created by reducing the final 50% of the deformity. The reduction maneuver entails potential stretching

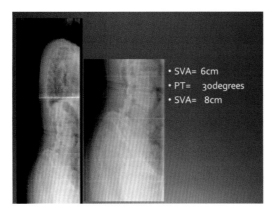

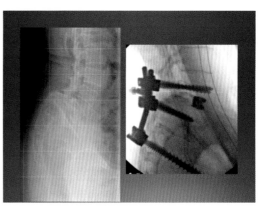

- SVA= 6cm
- PT= 30degrees
- SVA= 8cm

a

Fig. 13.5 (a,b) A 12-year-old girl presents with high-grade dysplastic spondylolisthesis with back pain, sagittal imbalance, and bilateral hamstring[23] tightness with tension signs. She had lumbopelvic and global spinal imbalance, and was type 6 on the Labelle classification. She underwent a deformity reduction with interbody fixation from a posterior approach. The reduction was achieved by mobilization of the L5 vertebra with a wide posterior-based annulotomy at L5-S1, an osteotomy across the sacral dome, and reduction of L5 on S1 using reduction screws, followed by placement of the interbody cage for segmental stabilization.

of the chronically displaced L5 nerve root in the anteroposterior (AP) and craniocaudal directions as the L5 body is reduced on the S1 end plate. The incidence of postoperative neurologic injuries after reduction is highly variable, with published reports of deficits ranging from 0 to 75%. Transient neurologic deficits are usually more common than reported in the literature, because most often only serious deficits are reported. Strategies to mitigate neurologic deficit include complete decompression of the L5 nerve roots and the use of intraoperative neuromonitoring such as electromyogram (EMG), motor evoked potentials (MEPs), and direct stimulation of the nerve, which is especially important during reduction to provide feedback to the surgeon, so as to perform reduction only when indicated and only to the extent needed to restore spinal balance.[24]

At the University of California, San Francisco, author S.H.B. utilizes high-density MEP to assess the L5 motor units and uses multimodal neuromonitoring to assess the L5 nerve function with high sensitivity and specificity. In the experience of author Y.M.G., most of the deficits occur in cases in which a reduction is attempted beyond grade II, and special emphasis is placed on tracking the nerve and ensuring that it feels and looks uncompressed throughout its tract. Based on anecdotal observations, correction of the lumbosacral kyphosis seems to be less associated with L5 nerve deficit compared with the translational reduction of the listhesis.

Chapter Summary

Dysplastic high-grade spondylolisthesis is an important and complex pathology in the pediatric patient with back pain. Patients with dysplastic high-grade spondylolisthesis have significant disability as measured by self-reported health assessments. Reduction of lumbopelvic deformity and realignment of the global balance of the spine is useful to improve the health status of patients with high-grade dysplastic deformity. The failure to reduce lumbopelvic parameters and global imbalance may become an apparent disability in adults. Patients with an imbalanced pelvis or imbalanced spine, that is types 5 and 6 in the Labelle classification, benefit from a partial reduction with transosseous stabilization and strut graft or with interbody fusion. This is based on the data suggesting that patients with high-grade spondylolisthesis and an imbalanced spine or pelvis have a poorer HRQOL, but this needs further corroboration with randomized clinic studies correlating the change in HRQOL with the change in radiographic parameters preoperatively and postoperatively.

Reduction of the listhesis can be achieved with a posterior-based decompression, sacral dome osteotomy, and reduction, or with combined anterior- and posterior-based procedures.

◆ Reduction improves the biomechanical stability of the L5-S1 interspace, the fusion rate, and the impact of the deformity on the patient's health.
◆ Treatment options include in situ fusion, posterior-based reduction, anterior shortening, and posterior-based fixation. In situ fusion is most useful in patients with a balanced pelvis and spine (type 4 deformity). Partial reduction with fusion is most useful for a type 5 deformity. More complete reduction of the lumbosacral alignment and the global spinal alignment is most useful in patients with a type 6 deformity.

Pearls

◆ It is important to differentiate dysplastic spondylolisthesis from other etiologies of spondylolisthesis.
◆ Recognition of the degree of dysplastic changes and the deficiency in the posterior elements is important for preoperative planning.
◆ Patients with spinopelvic imbalance are classified as types 5 and 6 in the Scoliosis Research Society (SRS)/Labelle classification and are candidates for reduction of the lumbopelvic malalignment and restoration of global spinal balance.

Pitfalls

◆ Failure to obtain full length films to assess the global alignment and spinal balance.
◆ Failure to understand the importance of reduction when indicated.
◆ Failure to decompress the L5 nerve roots completely when reduction is attempted, and failure to recognize excessive tension on the L5 roots with motor evoked potentials to detect possible postoperative radiculopathy.

References

Five Must-Read References

1. Herbiniaux G. Traite sur divers accouchemens laborleux et sur les polypes de la matrice. Bruxelles: J. L. DeBoubers; 1782
2. Wiltse LL, Newman PH, Macnab I. Classification of spondylolisis and spondylolisthesis. Clin Orthop Relat Res 1976;117:23–29
3. Wiltse LL. Etiology of spondylolisthesis. Clin Orthop 1957;10:48–60
4. Meyerding H. Spondylolisthesis as an etiologic factor in backache. JAMA 1938;111:1971–1976
5. Meyerding HW. Spondylolisthesis. J Bone Joint Surg. 1931;13:39–48
6. Wiltse LL, Winter RB. Terminology and measurement of spondylolisthesis. J Bone Joint Surg Am 1983;65: 768–772
7. Marchetti PG, Bartolozzi P. Classification of spondylolisthesis as a guideline for treatment. In: Bridwell KH, DeWald RL, eds. Textbook of Spinal Surgery, 2nd ed. Philadelphia: Lippincott-Raven; 1997:1211–1254
8. Mac-Thiong JM, Duong L, Parent S, et al. Reliability of the Spinal Deformity Study Group classification of lumbosacral spondylolisthesis. Spine 2012;37:E95– E102
9. Hresko MT, Labelle H, Roussouly P, Berthonnaud E. Classification of high-grade spondylolistheses based

on pelvic version and spine balance: possible rationale for reduction. Spine 2007;32:2208–2213
10. Labelle H, Roussouly P, Berthonnaud E, Dimnet J, O'Brien M. The importance of spino-pelvic balance in L5-s1 developmental spondylolisthesis: a review of pertinent radiologic measurements. Spine 2005;30 (6, Suppl):S27–S34
11. Glassman SD, Bridwell K, Dimar JR, Horton W, Berven S, Schwab F. The impact of positive sagittal balance in adult spinal deformity. Spine 2005;30:2024–2029
12. Roussouly P, Gollogly S, Berthonnaud E, Labelle H, Weidenbaum M. Sagittal alignment of the spine and pelvis in the presence of L5-S1 isthmic lysis and low-grade spondylolisthesis. Spine 2006;31:2484–2490
13. Poussa M, Remes V, Lamberg T, et al. Treatment of severe spondylolisthesis in adolescence with reduction or fusion in situ: long-term clinical, radiologic, and functional outcome. Spine 2006;31:583–590, discussion 591–592
14. Ruf M, Koch H, Melcher RP, Harms J. Anatomic reduction and monosegmental fusion in high-grade developmental spondylolisthesis. Spine 2006;31:269–274
15. Boxall D, Bradford DS, Winter RB, Moe JH. Management of severe spondylolisthesis in children and adolescents. J Bone Joint Surg Am 1979;61:479–495

16. Bohlman HH, Cook SS. One-stage decompression and posterolateral and interbody fusion for lumbosacral spondyloptosis through a posterior approach. Report of two cases. J Bone Joint Surg Am 1982;64:415–418

17. Smith JA, Deviren V, Berven S, Kleinstueck F, Bradford DS. Clinical outcome of trans-sacral interbody fusion after partial reduction for high-grade l5-S1 spondylolisthesis. Spine 2001;26:2227–2234

18. Hart RA, Domes CM, Goodwin B, et al. High-grade spondylolisthesis treated using a modified Bohlman technique: results among multiple surgeons. J Neurosurg Spine 2014;20:523–530

19. Bradford EH, Lovett RW. Spondylolisthesis. Treatise Orthop Surg. 1905;3:385–388

20. Bradford DS, Boachie-Adjei O. Treatment of severe spondylolisthesis by anterior and posterior reduction and stabilization. A long-term follow-up study. J Bone Joint Surg Am 1990;72:1060–1066

21. Gaines RW. L5 vertebrectomy for the surgical treatment of spondyloptosis: thirty cases in 25 years. Spine 2005;30(6, Suppl):S66–S70

22. Lehmer SM, Steffee AD, Gaines RW Jr. Treatment of L5-S1 spondyloptosis by staged L5 resection with reduction and fusion of L4 onto S1 (Gaines procedure). Spine 1994;19:1916–1925

23. Phalen G, Dickson J. Spondylolisthesis and tight hamstrings. J Bone Joint Surg. 1961;43:505–512

24. Lieberman JA, Lyon R, Feiner J, Hu SS, Berven SH. The efficacy of motor evoked potentials in fixed sagittal imbalance deformity correction surgery. Spine 2008; 33:E414–E424

14

Kyphotic Deformity in the Pediatric Spine

Avery L. Buchholz, John C. Quinn, Christopher I. Shaffrey,
Sigurd H. Berven, David W. Polly, Jr., and Justin S. Smith

⑳ Introduction

Kyphotic deformity in the pediatric spine may be caused by multiple disorders. The clinical presentation of kyphotic deformity varies depending on the age of the child, the severity of the curve at time of diagnosis, and the underlying cause. In many instances the spinal anomaly is just part of the problem in a globally affected patient, and other systems including neuromuscular disorders and intraspinal abnormalities may occur concordantly. It is important to understand the natural history of specific conditions that cause kyphotic deformity, the dynamics of growth in the developing spine, and axial skeletal biomechanics in order to determine the appropriate treatment. This chapter provides an overview of kyphotic deformity in the pediatric spine, and discusses the etiologies, concurrent pathologies, developmental patterns, and treatment.

Hyperkyphosis, sometimes referred to as round back or hunchback, is defined as a curve with abnormally increased posterior convex angulation. In contrast to scoliotic deformities, kyphotic deformities are more typically confined to one plane (sagittal). In the pediatric population, the etiologies are diverse, encompassing congenital anomalies, neuromuscular conditions, developmental disorders, skeletal dysplasia, infections, trauma, surgical sequela, and, more rarely, neoplastic processes. The most common kyphotic deformity in pediatric patients is Scheuermann kyphosis, which is the focus of this chapter. Other causes, including congenital anomalies and neuromuscular disorders, are also discussed. The risk of pediatric kyphosis progression is dependent on the cause of the deformity, the severity of the deformity, and the growth remaining. Appropriate management of pediatric kyphosis requires an understanding of the natural history and the risk of progression.

⑳ Scheuermann Disease

Scheuermann disease is the most common cause of structural kyphosis in adolescents. Reports show an incidence of 0.4 to 8.0% in the general population, but the diagnosis is likely underreported, as it often goes unrecognized or is attributed to poor posture.[1] Originally described in 1921 by Holger Scheuermann,[2] the disease was identified as a rigid spinal kyphosis, differentiating it from the more correctable postural roundback. It was further characterized radiographically by Sorenson[3] as vertebral body wedging of greater than 5 degrees in at least three contiguous vertebrae, end plate irregularity, and the presence of Schmorl's nodes. A definitive distinction between abnormal kyphosis and pathognomonic signs of

Scheuermann disease may be difficult because the disease encompasses a broad spectrum of vertebral anomalies.[4]

The specific etiology of Scheuermann disease remains unclear. It was initially thought to result from avascular necrosis of the vertebral ring apophyses that leads to premature growth arrest and wedging.[5] Schmorl proposed an inherent weakness of the cartilaginous end plates. Various mechanical theories have also been proposed, implicating the anterior longitudinal ligament and anterior column pressure changes. Bracing has been advocated to relieve pain and reverse vertebral wedging, giving support to a mechanical etiology.[6] Murray et al[1] have questioned the long-term utility of bracing in their long-term follow-up study. No high-quality studies (level 1 or 2) support or refute the evidence for bracing or casting. In addition, Scheuermann disease has been associated with endocrine abnormalities, inflammatory disease, and neuromuscular disorders. Juvenile osteoporosis may also play a role.[7,8] Varying degrees of scoliosis are seen radiographically in one third of patients with Scheuermann disease. Isthmic spondylolisthesis has also been reported more commonly in patients with Scheuermann disease and may be a cause of low back pain.[9]

Scheuermann disease is commonly detected at puberty. Often it is ignored or dismissed by parents and teachers who attribute it to poor posture. It is rare in patients younger than 10 years of age, with the typical presentation in the late juvenile period, and the more severe form appearing between the ages of 12 and 16 years.[4] Scheuermann disease and postural kyphosis can be differentiated by the rigidity of the kyphotic deformity. Trunk extension will produce deformity correction in those with postural kyphosis, whereas there is little correction in the rigid Scheuermann kyphosis. Patients with Scheuermann disease may also suffer from contractures of the pectoralis muscles, hip flexors, and hamstrings.

The effect of Scheuermann disease on health-related quality of life has been variable. In a study comparing health-related quality of life in patients with Scheuermann kyphosis to patients with adolescent idiopathic scoliosis and normal controls, Lonner et al[10] demonstrated that patients with Scheuermann kyphosis had more impairment in every domain of the Scoliosis Research Society Outcomes Questionnaire (SRS-22) including pain, function, mental health, and self image. In contrast, Ristolainen et al[11] evaluated 80 adults with untreated Scheuermann kyphosis, and concluded that affected adults had a higher risk of back pain compared with controls. In addition, the patients with untreated Scheuermann kyphosis reported lower quality of life and poorer general health than did controls. The risk of disabilities affecting the performance of activities of the daily living was high in patients than in controls. However, among the patients there was no correlation between the degree of kyphosis and self-reported quality of life or health status or back pain.

The clinical presentation of the disease may vary from minimal or no symptoms in some patients to significant disability in others.[1] Symptoms, when present, encompass nonradiating pain, physical disability, decreased range of motion, weakness of the back, restrictive lung disease, and hamstring tightness, leading to decreased participation in physical activity in employment and in athletics.[7] Adolescents typically are more concerned with self-image but may report neck pain, back pain, and fatigue as well. In these patients, pain is typically below the apex of the curve in the paraspinal musculature, which may be a result of the increased incidence of lumbosacral spondylolisthesis, spondylosis, disk degeneration, and scoliosis in patients with Scheuermann disease. Spondylolysis in particular has been reported in up to 50% of these patients.[9] Neural symptoms are rare in pediatric patients with Scheuermann disease, although paraparesis has been reported. When present, neural symptoms are often associated with herniated thoracic disks, spinal stenosis, dural cysts, or extreme kyphotic deformity with tenting of the spinal cord over the apex of the deformity.[6] There are reports of acute cord compression due to traumatic disk herniation as well as other reports of intraoperative herniations during kyphosis correction. To summarize, patients with Scheuermann kyphosis may be neurologically intact, although with varying degrees of reserve and significant anterior displacement of the spinal cord within the canal, possibly making them more vulnerable to acute neurologic deterioration from typically benign lesions such as disk bulges, ventral compression, or disruptions of blood flow to the spinal cord.[12]

Thoracic kyphosis in unaffected populations is variable, and typically ranges from 20 to 40 degrees using the Cobb method on erect lateral radiograph.[13] Scheuermann disease is best seen by evaluating standing full spine lateral radiographs.[14] Diagnostic criteria based on Sorenson include the presence of > 5 degrees of anterior wedging in at least three consecutive vertebrae at the apex of the kyphotic deformity. Patients typically also have narrowed disk spaces, endplate irregularities, and Schmorl's nodes (**Fig. 14.1**). A radiograph obtained with the patient hyperextended over a bolster demonstrates the degree of stiffness of the kyphotic curve. Two different curve patterns have been described in Scheuermann disease.[15] The more common pattern is thoracic, with an apex at T8-T9 that is usually quite rigid and balanced. The less common pattern is thoracolumbar, with an apex at T10-T11 that is normally flexible and frequently unbalanced[15] (**Fig. 14.2**). If neurologic findings are present, additional evaluation by magnetic resonance imaging (MRI) is generally indicated. This imaging may detect myelopathy or cord compression, thoracic disk herniation, and other subtleties that which may alter the treatment approach. MRI may also be helpful in evaluating the neural elements in intact patients and can assist in surgical planning.

Treatment

The treatment of Scheuermann disease is primarily nonoperative, and includes anti-inflammatory medications, exercise, bracing, and casting. In a skeletally immature patient with a mild deformity, routine evaluation with radiographs every 6 months is recommended. Once the diagnosis has been made, it is important to maintain close observation until skeletal maturity. Adolescents with kyphosis of less than 60 degrees are typically treated with physical therapy and exercise programs until skeletal maturity. Exercise and physical therapy are useful to treat associated back pain and to improve muscle tone and posture, though these modalities have not been shown to alter progression of the deformity.

Bracing and casting have been effectively used in patients with kyphotic deformities and sufficient growth (age < 12 or RIser grade 0–2) remaining. The initial report by Bradford et al[16]

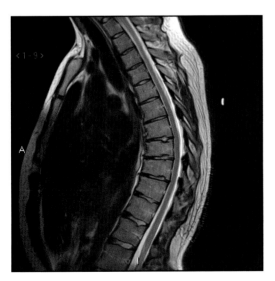
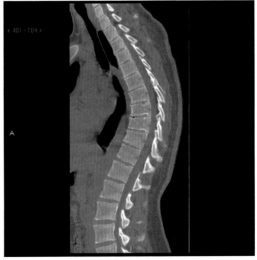

b

Fig. 14.1 (a) Preoperative magnetic resonance imaging (MRI) and **(b)** computed tomography (CT) scan showing Scheuermann disease diagnostic criteria including end-plate irregularities, Schmorl nodes, and 5 degrees of kyphosis in more than three sequential levels.

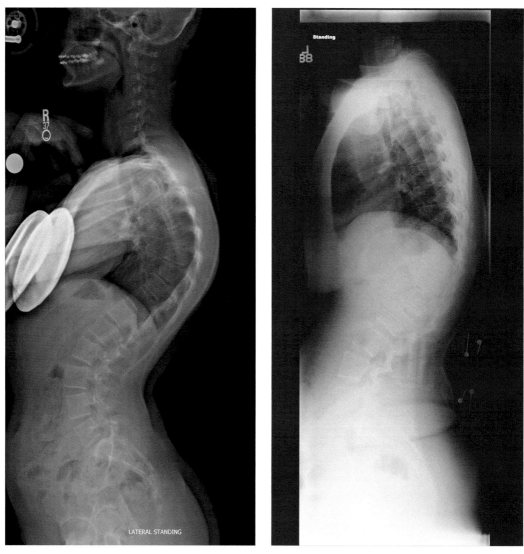

a

Fig. 14.2 Two types of curve seen in Scheuermann disease. **(a)** The more common curve type with a T8–T9 apex. **(b)** The less common type with a T11 apex.

demonstrated a 40% decrease in mean thoracic kyphosis, and a 35% decrease in mean lumbar lordosis after 34 months of bracing. Gutowski and Renshaw[17] reported on the use of the Boston and Milwaukee braces in a group of 75 patients. Compliant patients had 35% improvement in the Milwaukee brace compared with 27% in the Boston brace. Milwaukee brace treatment consistently improved kyphosis by ~ 50% during the active phase of treatment. Skeletally immature adolescents with progressive kyphosis > 45 degrees or with curves of up to 65 degrees should be considered for a trial

of bracing. Prior to considering brace treatment, a hyperextension X-ray over a bolster is helpful to assess the flexibility of the deformity. Patients with at least 40% passive correction of curves measuring between 50 and 75 degrees often respond well to bracing. Those with > 75 degrees of curvature respond less favorably to bracing, and surgical intervention should be considered for these patients. Murray et al[1] suggest that bracing is not effective in the long term for Scheuermann kyphosis.

Surgery in Scheuermann disease may be indicated in patients with kyphosis > 75 degrees, in patients with kyphosis > 55 degrees and with pain that is unresponsive to nonoperative care, patients with progression of curve despite bracing, those with an unacceptable appearance, and in rare instances of neurologic deficit. Cardiopulmonary compromise is not usually associated with thoracic hyperkyphosis. Surgery is generally not indicated in skeletally immature patients with kyphosis < 75 degrees unless their symptomatic deformity is not responsive to nonoperative care. Other factors to consider are patient age and the location and shape of the kyphosis. The goals of surgical treatment are to prevent curve progression, improve pain, restore sagittal alignment, and improve cosmetic appearance.[18]

The surgical techniques for the treatment of Scheuermann kyphosis have evolved over several decades and include posterior-only, combined anterior and posterior, and anterior-alone procedures. Traditionally, anterior release combined with posterior fusion had been used to treat severe rigid deformities that did not correct to < 50 degrees on hyperextension X-rays. Modern pedicle screw instrumentation systems have improved the ability to control and realign the spine, reducing the need for anterior release and making posterior-only approaches sufficient for most cases. Posterior-only procedures enable posterior column shortening via segmental compression, which may be combined with multilevel posterior column or, less frequently, three-column osteotomies for correction of large deformities.

In North America, the terms *Smith-Petersen osteotomy* and *Ponte osteotomy* are often used incorrectly to describe the same technique. This can cause confusion. To overcome this difficulty, we will refer to them collectively as a posterior column osteotomy (PCO) throughout the chapter. The Smith-Petersen osteotomy (SPO) was initially described for use in the lumbar spine, and it consisted of a narrow resection of lumbar facet joints with detachment of the ligamentum flavum from the inferior margin of the lamina and inferior articular process. There was no resection of the lamina in the original description, and correction was gained at a single level with osteoclasis of the anterior column and anterior column distraction.[19] When SPOs are used in thoracic defor-

mity, it is generally to obtain flexibility in stiff curves such as those seen with ankylosing spondylitis. Flexibility and kyphosis correction is then obtained by opening the anterior disk spaces with lengthening of the anterior column.

The Ponte osteotomy consists of complete resection of the thoracic facet joints and wide lamina resection with complete removal of ligamentum flavum.[20] Correction is dependent on the mobility of the intervertebral disk, with distraction of the anterior column and compression of the posterior disk. The absence of anterior column disruption preserves the immediate and long-term load-sharing capacity and the stability of correction. Current recommendations are for bilateral pedicle screw fixation at every instrumented level, with PCOs in the thoracic and lumbar spine. Surgical techniques obtain correction by combining anterior lengthening through the intervertebral disk and posterior shortening by PCO of the spine.

The PCO enables closure and shortening of the posterior elements, resulting in decreased kyphosis. We prefer to first prepare all implant sites prior to the osteotomy. This preserves the anatomy so that proper screw trajectories can be obtained and the risk of neurologic injury is decreased with no dura exposed. In the PCO, the spinous process is removed entirely. A high-speed drill is used to cut a fracture line across the lamina and bilateral pars. Osteotomes and Capener gouge instruments are used to fracture the remaining pars/lamina bone, with this segment generally removed as a solid piece. Any remaining bone of the inferior articulating process is removed with a narrow Leksell rongeur, and the superior articulating process is carefully removed with Kerrison rongeurs, being sure to leave no bone or soft tissue that may be capable of causing foraminal obstruction during compression. Any remaining ligamentum flavum or lamina causing stenosis may then be removed, being careful to maintain a segment of intact lamina for stability and for a posterior fusion surface. This resection of bone can result in 5 to 7 degrees of correction when compressed posteriorly[20] (**Fig. 14.3**).

Geck et al[20] reviewed 17 consecutive patients undergoing posterior-only pedicle screw instrumentation with PCO, and reported excellent

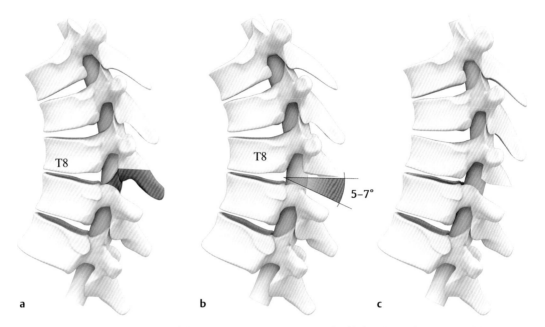

Fig. 14.3 **(a)** Sagittal illustration of thoracic spine with bone to be removed in posterior column osteotomy highlighted red. **(b)** Sagittal illustration of thoracic spine with PCO complete and potential correction highlighted in red. **(c)** Sagittal illustration of thoracic spine after one level PCO and kyphosis correction complete.

correction compared with anterior-posterior technique controls. Lonner et al[21] also compared anterior-posterior and posterior-only procedures. Patients undergoing anterior-posterior were noted to have more overall complications (23.8% versus 5.5%) and an increased rate of junctional kyphosis (32% versus 4%), although they were noted to have decreased loss of correction (3.2 versus 6.4 degrees). The groups had similar reoperation rates (5.1%) due to symptomatic junctional kyphosis.

Treatment of Scheuermann disease should aim to correct the kyphosis to the high normal range of thoracic kyphosis (40 to 50 degrees). Overcorrection of a kyphotic deformity can lead to neurologic complications, postoperative sagittal malalignment, and proximal junctional kyphosis (PJK). Lowe and Kasten[22] recommended that no more than 50% of the preoperative kyphosis be corrected, and that the final kyphosis should never be less than 40 degrees. This is achieved through two techniques: segmentally applied and apically directed com-

pression forces, and cantilever reduction. With cantilever reduction two 5.5- or 6.0-mm rods are contoured to an anticipated kyphosis, inserted into the pedicle screws proximal to the apex, and cantilevered into the distal implants. This technique has been implicated in junctional kyphosis, with the force concentrated on either end of the construct. Apical compression techniques use multisegment fixation and compression toward the apex to reduce the kyphosis. This has the advantage of spreading out reduction forces to the entire construct rather than being concentrated at junctional levels. A review by Denis et al[23] found the majority of Scheuermann correction was achieved by a combination of cantilever and apical compression techniques. They found no difference in the rate of PJK between any of the techniques used. Both hooks and pedicle screws are safe and efficacious, but most surgeons prefer the mechanical advantage afforded by pedicle screws in deformity correction.

We have found success reducing strain on proximal and distal screw foundations seen in cantilever loading by using temporary apical cantilever rods and sequential reduction of the correction rod. Final full-length rods are then secured when the kyphotic spine is almost fully corrected. We prefer to lock the proximal three or four screws in place with no corrective force, and cantilever them into the distal segments. Although improvement in the instrumentation enables more effective force application to the spine for deformity correction, the ultimate success of the correction relies on the effectiveness of the release.

It is rare for Scheuermann kyphosis to need release beyond PCO, but in some instances a three-column osteotomy may be necessary, which may include a vertebral column resection (VCR) or less commonly a pedicle subtraction osteotomy (PSO). Vertebral column resection is reserved for use in the thoracic or thoracolumbar spine for the treatment of sharp or angular kyphotic deformity, fixed kyphotic segments, or congenital malformations. Advantages include the potential for dramatic correction in all three dimensions and overall shortening of the vertebral column, which help to relieve tension on the anterior neurovascular structures. Correction up to 45 degrees in the sagittal plane has been reported.[24] VCR involves complete resection of all posterior elements at the level of the VCR in addition to complete removal of the vertebral body and adjacent rostral and caudal intervertebral disks. In most cases, an anterior fusion is performed with structural support via an anterior cage that enables preservation of the anterior column height, re-creation of the lordosis, and enhanced correction (**Fig. 14.4**). VCR remains the most powerful method of three-dimensional deformity correction; however, the technique poses the greatest technical challenge and the greatest risk to the patient in terms of possible neurologic injury, operative time, blood loss, and potential morbidity.

Pedicle subtraction osteotomies are seldom used in the thoracic spine because wedging of the thoracic vertebra limit the height of the anterior column, and therefore the potential for correction. However, in the lumbar spine, or if there is sufficient anterior vertebral height, a wedge resection or pedicle subtraction may be a useful technique for deformity correction. The procedure is typically associated with shortening of the posterior column without lengthening the anterior column. A PSO requires removal of all posterior elements at the level of correction, including the pedicles and superior and inferior adjacent facet joints. A posterior wedge of bone is then removed from the vertebral body, including the entire posterior and lateral vertebral body walls, to enable

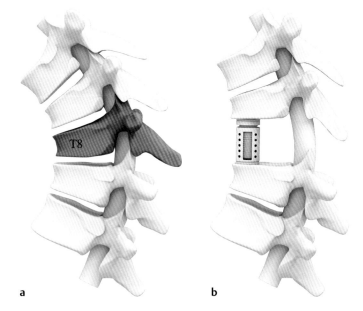

a   b

Fig. 14.4 (a) Sagittal illustration of thoracic spine with kyphotic vertebral segment to be removed in vertebral column resection (VCR) highlighted red. **(b)** Sagittal illustration of thoracic spine after VCR and anteriorly placed vertebral body cage with kyphosis correction.

osteotomy closure. This results in bone-on-bone approximation with a high rate of healing. We have found that a PSO can achieve up to 35 degrees of correction (**Fig. 14.5**). PSOs are again preferred below the level of the conus, but can be performed in the thoracic spine, although with increased risk.[25] With an extended PSO the bony resection extends cranially to include the rostral intervertebral disk. The vertebral end plate is then closed directly onto the cancellous osteotomy wedge or the PSO. An interbody spacer can be placed in the middle or anterior third of the disk space to be used as a fulcrum, obtaining the same correction with less compromise of the neural structures. Again, PSO is rarely indicated in the thoracic spine but may be considered for fixed thoracic deformity or thoracolumbar congenital malformations.

The selection of the appropriate level for instrumentation and fusion is an important consideration in the treatment of Scheuermann disease. It is important to extend the fusion over the entire length of the kyphotic deformity. Failure to do so may result in PJK or distal junctional kyphosis (DJK). Junctional kyphosis most often is a result of junctional ligamentous disruption, too much deformity correction, and failure to incorporate appropriate vertebra. Most surgeons agree that the upper limit of the fusion must be the proximal end vertebra in the measured kyphosis, or to the level of the first lordotic disk.[22] For high- and midthoracic apex deformities, the upper-instrumented vertebra is typically T2 or T3. Fusions short of the proximal end vertebra and disruption of the junctional ligaments are the main risk factors for PJK. In a study of 40 patients in whom the fusion incorporated the proximal end vertebra, three had disruption of junctional ligaments and all three developed PJK.[23]

There has been debate regarding the distal extend of fusion. Some authors advocate extending fusion to the first lordotic vertebra (FLV). Denis et al[23] assessed 67 patients who had correction of Scheuermann kyphosis. Eight patients developed DJK, with seven of them having fusion short of the FLV. Other authors advocate extending the fusion to the second lordotic vertebra. Poolman et al[26] reported on a

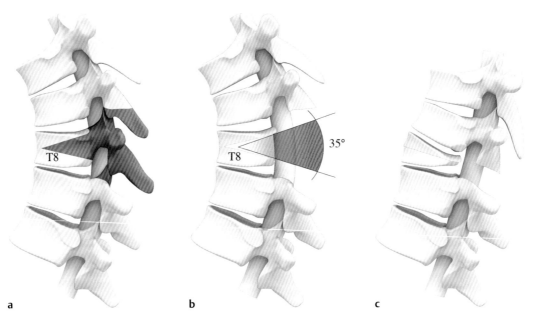

a b c

Fig. 14.5 **(a)** Sagittal illustration of thoracic spine with bone to be removed in pedicle subtraction osteotomy (PSO) highlighted red. **(b)** Sagittal illustration of thoracic spine after PSO with potential kyphosis correction in red. **(c)** Sagitttal illustration of thoracic spine after PSO with correction achieved noting bone on bone contact at PSO site.

series of patients with no DJK when the second lordotic vertebra was incorporated into the fusion.

More recently the concepts of sagittal stable vertebra (SSV) and its relationship to the lowest instrumented vertebra (LIV) and FLV have become important considerations. The SSV is the most proximal vertebra touched by the posterior sacral vertical line (PSVL), with the PSVL being a vertical line from the posterior-superior corner of the sacrum on a lateral upright radiograph. When the LIV includes the SSV, the fusion mass will be centered over the sacrum in the sagittal plane, achieving improved global balance. Cho et al[27] reported a series of 24 consecutive patients with no DJK when the SSV was included in the distal fusion. To maintain global sagittal alignment after surgery, both the proximal and distal ends of the fusion should be within the center of gravity. This equates to a fusion incorporating the upper end of kyphosis and SSV distally. The disadvantage of incorporating the SSV is that the fusion level may be one segment longer distal to the FLV, with loss of a mobile segment. Another important consideration is the postoperative lumbopelvic mismatch. Following correction of the thoracic spine, there is simultaneous reduction in lumbar lordosis. Patients with a high pelvic incidence should undergo a smaller thoracic kyphosis reduction to prevent excessive loss of lumbar lordosis. Nasto et al[28] reported a higher incidence of PJK in patients with significant lumbopelvic mismatch. Overall, distal fusion including the FLV but not the SSV is not appropriate in all patients, with distal junctional problems developing more often in patients with fusion to the FLV rather than the SSV. Selection of fusion levels remains an important and challenging aspect of kyphosis surgery, and overcorrection should be avoided.

With Scheuermann disease there are some additional complications to consider. Lonner et al[29] documented a comparison of Scheuermann kyphosis correction with adolescent idiopathic scoliosis (AIS) correction, and found Scheuermann patients were 3.9 times more likely to have a major complication. Scheuermann patients were also significantly more likely to undergo a second operation and experience infections. The prolonged operative time, anatomic variation, and lower incidence of operative Scheuermann patients have all been proposed as reasons for increased complications in Scheuermann disease compared with AIS patients.

Case Examples

Case 1

A 14-year-old pre-menarche girl presents with worsening kyphosis over the past 2 years and increased concern over appearance. She reports low back pain with prolonged sitting or standing but denies any numbness, tingling, or radicular pain. She continues to be active playing soccer and volleyball. MRI shows no central canal stenosis but anterior wedging of T7, T8, and T9 with associated disk changes at T7-T8 and T8–T9, representing Scheuermann disease. Upright standing lateral films show 90 degrees of kyphosis from T4 to T11 with 63 degrees of kyphosis in the supine position.

The patient undergoes posterior T2–L2 pedicle screw instrumentation with PCOs from T4 to T11 and placement of a Mersilene tether from T1 to a T5–T6 cross-link. The Mersilene tape is tied from the spinous process proximal to the upper-instrumented level to the cross-link and tightened using distraction. This is performed in an attempt to reduce proximal junctional kyphosis (**Fig. 14.6**).

Postoperatively, the patient does well with improved posture and decreased low back pain. Her T4–T11 kyphosis measures 30 degrees.

Case 2

A 27-year-old man underwent previous anterior release and T4-L2 posterior fusion at age 18 for Scheuermann kyphosis. Patient suffered postoperative infection and ultimately had instrumentation removed 6 months after surgery, with treatment in a brace since that time. The patient now presents with continued back pain and progressive kyphosis. He has no leg numbness, tingling, weakness or radicular pain, or bowel or bladder issues. Standing lateral radiographs show thoracic kyphosis of 100 degrees.

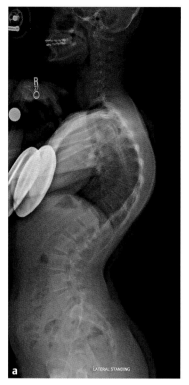
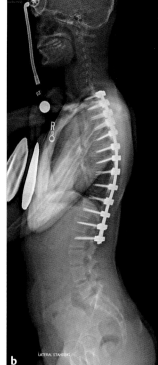
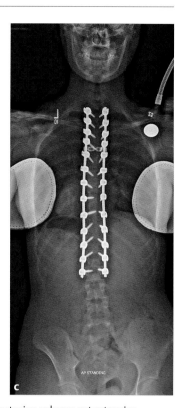

Fig. 14.6 **(a)** Preoperative standing sagittal radiograph in a patient with Scheuermann disease. **(b)** Postoperative sagittal radiograph showing correction of deformity with bilateral pedicle screws and multilevel posterior column osteotomies (PCOs). **(c)** Postoperative anteroposterior (AP) radiograph showing proper coronal alignment.

The patient undergoes posterior T2–L3 pedicle screw instrumentation and PCOs at T4–T5, T5–T6, T6–T7, T12-L1, and L1–L2, as well as T10 complete vertebral column resection with partial T9 vertebral column resection and a 15 × 30 mm interbody spacer (**Fig. 14.7**).

Postoperatively, the patient does well with significant improvement in back pain and correction of thoracic kyphosis to 50 degrees.

▊ Congenital Kyphosis

Congenital kyphosis results from early embryologic failure of segmentation or formation of one or multiple vertebral bodies. As with any spinal disorder arising during embryological formation, the heart, kidneys, trachea, esophagus, and gastrointestinal (GI) system need to be evaluated, as the association between congenital spine disorders and additional organ system abnormalities is well documented.[30,31] The classification of congenital kyphosis is relevant to the natural history, prognosis, and treatment of the deformity. Classically, congenital kyphosis has been grouped into three categories: type I, failure of formation; type II, failure of segmentation; and type III, mixed[32] (**Fig. 14.8**). This system was expanded to include those cases that are unable to be diagnosed radiographically: type IV, unclassifiable. A fifth and more severe type has been described and has been termed congenital dislocated spine.[33] Even in congenital cases it may be unusual for a deformity to be clinically evident at birth. These anomalies may also not be apparent on radiographs initially because of the incomplete ossification of the spine in the newborn.

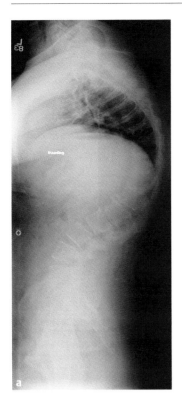 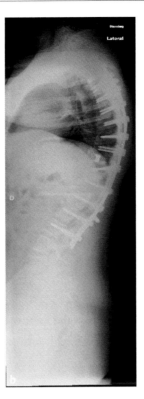

Fig. 14.7 **(a)** Preoperative standing sagittal radiograph in a patient with Scheuermann disease showing 100-degree thoracic kyphosis. **(b)** Post-operative standing sagittal radiograph showing thoracic kyphosis of 50 degrees and proper sagittal balance.

Defects of vertebral-body segmentation	Defects of vertebral-body formation		Mixed anomalies
Partial	**Anterior and unilateral aplasia**	**Anterior and median aplasia**	
Anterior unsegmented bar	**Posterolateral quadrant vertebra**	**Butterfly vertebra**	**Anterolateral bar and contralateral quadrant vertebra**
Complete	**Anterior aplasia**	**Anterior hypoplasia**	
Block vertebra	**Posterior hemivertebra**	**Wedged vertebra**	

Fig. 14.8 The classification of congenital deformity. Reproduced with permission from McMaster MJ, Singh H. Natural history of congenital kyhosis and kyphoscoliosis. A study of one hundred and twelve patients. JBJS 1999;81:1367–1383.

In general, the natural history of congenital kyphosis is dependent on the pathoanatomy, patient age, and the severity of the deformity. Congenital kyphosis may have significant progression; deformity may become severe, and neural deficit may develop. Curves may occur in the spine at any location, although the thoracolumbar region is the most common. Progression is variable but typically occurs with growth of the spine and is accelerated between the ages of 1 and 5 years and again at 10 years to skeletal maturity.[32] Type I anomalies, failure of formation, are most commonly seen, and, if progressive, can often lead to neurologic compromise. These lesions tend to produce sharp, angular deformity and thus can lead to acute angulation and compromise of the spinal cord. Type II anomalies, failure of segmentation, produce a smooth kyphosis and have no reported incidence of neurologic deterioration in the literature.[32] However, the rule of progressive curvature remains, and Mayfield et al[34] reported progression of up to 5 degrees per year for these anomalies. Type III anomalies tend to be the most progressive and severe. They have been reported to progress at a rate of 5 degrees per year prior to adolescence and 8 degrees per year during adolescence. They are associated with spastic paraparesis, and aggressive treatment is warranted.[33] Type IV anomalies, by definition, are severe, as they are unclassifiable by radiological evaluation. It is difficult to classify their natural history, given that most patients present with severe spinal deformities. Patients with congenital vertebral displacement tend to present in infancy with spinal deformity. Often this is associated with infantile paraplegia.[34]

Treatment

The management of congenital kyphosis centers on observation or operative treatments. Bracing has no role in congenital kyphosis.[32] The surgical treatment options vary, and similar to other pediatric deformities, depends on patient age, the type of deformity, the degree of curvature, and the presence or absence of neural findings. The use of spinal instrumentation has been shown to be safe and effective even in the youngest of patients.[35] In general, posterior-only arthrodesis is most effective in type I and III deformities. A solid posterior arthrodesis allows future anterior growth to take place. Current data suggest that patients younger than 5 years of age with a localized kyphosis < 50 degrees will be successfully treated with posterior arthrodesis alone.[35] Type II deformity has less potential for anterior growth and typically requires a circumferential approach or a three-column osteotomy. All congenital kyphosis types I, II, and III > 50 degrees in children younger than 5 years may also require a combined anterior and posterior approach or a posterior three-column osteotomy. Posterior-only approaches without three-column osteotomies are associated with a high rate of pseudarthrosis and poor correction in these patients. In patients over 5 years of age, an instrumented partial correction with PCO is acceptable. Complete correction is not necessary due to continued anterior–posterior growth differential. In patients over 10 years of age or with a Risser grade 2 to 3, there is not much anterior growth left, and a complete correction should be achieved. If correction is too great to achieve with PCO, a pedicle subtraction osteotomy or circumferential osteotomy should be considered. In all cases neurologic compression should be assessed and treated accordingly.

Case Example

A 4-year-old boy with congenital kyphosis from the L2 hemivertebra presents with regression of milestones, including loss of bladder control and decreased ability to ambulate due to compression on the conus of the spinal cord. On exam, the patient walks with a swayed back and has a deformity that partially corrects under traction when he is lifted off the ground. He has normal sensation and muscle tone in the upper and lower extremities.

The patient undergoes an L2 hemivertebra resection and T12–L3 posterior instrumented spinal fusion. The deformity is reduced with cantilever 4.5-mm rods. The patient is kept in a thoracolumbar support brace postoperative for 6 weeks. At 3 weeks, the patient's ambulation has improved and urinary retention is resolved. Brace weaning is then initiated (**Fig. 14.9**).

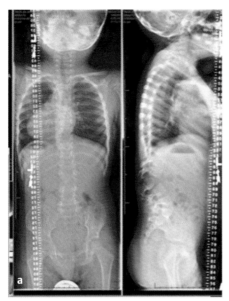
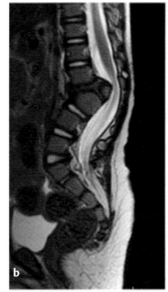
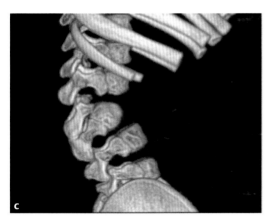
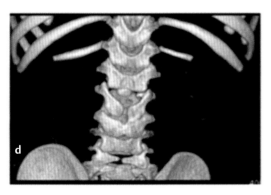
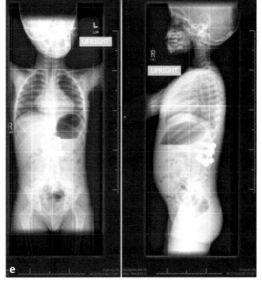

Fig. 14.9 A 4-year-old boy with congenital kyphosis from the L2 hemivertebra. **(a)** AP and lateral standing films showing the L2 hemivertebra. **(b–d)** MRI and three-dimensional CT reconstruction showing L2 hemivertebra. **(e)** T12–L3 posterior spinal fusion (PSF) postoperative AP and lateral standing films at 3 months' follow-up.

▥ Neuromuscular Disease

Neuromuscular kyphosis and scoliosis often develop secondary to neuromuscular imbalance, trauma, disease, birth defects, and syndromes. The deformity develops because of the neurologic or muscular disease but progresses because of the child's growth. Due to associated pathology, these patients present unique challenges to medical and surgical teams. Although brace treatment may not prevent kyphosis, it may slow the progression and allow for spinal growth before the spinal fusion. It may also help with function and allow physical therapy to maximize physical activity prior to surgery. Intrathecal baclofen (ITB) pumps have also been used in these patients to reduce spasticity and improve function. There have been reports of increased progression of deformity after the use of intrathecal baclofen pumps, but generally they are beneficial, and surgeons should anticipate their patients having an ITB pump at some point during the treatment process.[36] The severe spasticity seen in these patients can undo the most secure instrumentation if not controlled adequately.

Additional challenges associated with the surgical care of these patients include respiratory and cardiac function, nutritional issues, wound care, contractures, and anatomic considerations. Spinal deformity can impact respiratory mechanics, and the underlying pathology itself may impair ventilation. Cardiac myopathies may be common in certain neuromuscular diseases. Patients with neuromuscular disease often have nutritional issues with poor oral intake and gastroesophageal reflux. They may also have high metabolic demands. During the months preceding surgery, particular attention should be paid to nutritional management. This may involve nocturnal feeding with nasogastric tubes or supplementation with gastrostomy tubes. Preoperatively, there may be recurrent pressure ulcers, which should be addressed. Incisions require close monitoring postoperatively. Upper and lower extremity contractures can make positioning in surgery difficult, whereas hip and knee contractures may make addressing pelvic obliquity difficult.[37] The spine affected by neuromuscular disease often also has significant pedicle pleomorphism and laminar abnormalities.

Pelvic obliquity can originate from leg length inequality, contractures, and spinal deformity. A progressive pelvic obliquity with an unbalanced spine adversely affects sitting balance, comfort, and quality of life. The main goal of surgical treatment is to provide a solid and aligned spinopelvic unit in both planes to provide firm sitting balance.[38] Traditionally, extending a fusion to the pelvis was not recommended in ambulatory patients with pelvic obliquity; however, the literature in recent decades has found no difference in functional status in the long term.[39] Galveston iliac fixation enables the correction of pelvic obliquity and provides a stable point over which to balance the head and shoulders. In patients who are ambulatory, iliac screw fixation can add strength and support to the lumbosacral fusion.[40] Combined sacral and iliac fixation, spinopelvic transiliac fixation, and bilateral S1 and S2 screws have all been shown to provide excellent fixation and surgical outcomes. Surgical management of these patients continues to evolve with improved spinal and pelvic fixation.

▥ Postlaminectomy

In the pediatric population, a strong correlation between multilevel laminectomy and postlaminectomy spinal deformity has been demonstrated. This has mainly been observed in the cervical and thoracic spine. The reported incidence of laminectomy-related spinal kyphosis ranges from 33 to 100%. To reduce the risk of kyphosis, many authors advocate the use of laminoplasty. Laminoplasty is said to offer the required exposure and decompression of the spinal canal while maintaining spinal stability and the integrity of the posterior spinal elements. Therefore, laminoplasty is the recommended treatment of choice for skeletally immature pediatric patients with intraspinal mass lesions of the thoracic spine.[41]

▥ Chapter Summary

There are multiple causes of kyphotic deformity in the pediatric spine. A thorough history and physical exam as well as radiographic analysis will usually delineate the etiology. The most common causes include Scheuermann disease, congenital anomalies, neuromuscular disease, and postlaminectomy. Regardless of the etiology, surgical intervention is generally indicated in those with intractable pain and functional limitations, progressive deformity, and neurologic impairment.

Pearls

- ◆ Understanding the natural history of disease and the risk of any progressive kyphosis is a priority in deciding on operative care or observation.
- ◆ Level selection and instrumentation should at least extend over the entire length of the kyphosis (end-to-end vertebrae), and in Scheuermann's kyphosis the distal instrumented vertebra should be bisected by stable sagittal vertebra.

- ◆ For Scheuermann's kyphosis, the goal is to correct by 50% or to high normal values for kyphosis (40 to 45 degrees). Excessive correction of kyphosis may lead to junctional kyphosis.
- ◆ Congenital kyphosis needs to be viewed as a condition in which progression is the rule, deformity may become severe, and neurologic deficit is a possibility.

Pitfall

- ◆ The high risk of neural complications associated with correction of kyphosis may be related to vascular insufficiency or to ventral column compression from disk material or osteophytes. Preoperative MRI may be useful to identify ventral cord compression. Neuromonitoring is important for intraoperative safety.

Acknowledgment

We thank Emma Vought, MS, CMI, for her work on the illustrations and contribution to this chapter.

References
Five Must-Read References

1. Murray PM, Weinstein SL, Spratt KF. The natural history and long-term follow-up of Scheuermann kyphosis. J Bone Joint Surg Am 1993;75:236–248
2. Scheuermann HW. Kyphosis dorsalis juvenilis. Orthop Chir 1921;41:305
3. Sorenson KH. Scheuermann Juvenile Kyphosis. Clinical Appearances, Radiography, Aetiology, and Prognosis. Copenhagen: Munksgaard; 1964
4. Wenger DR, Frick SL. Scheuermann kyphosis. Spine 1999;24:2630–2639
5. Halal F, Gledhill RB, Fraser C. Dominant inheritance of Scheuermann's juvenile kyphosis. Am J Dis Child 1978;132:1105–1107
6. Tribus CB. Scheuermann's kyphosis in adolescents and adults: diagnosis and management. J Am Acad Orthop Surg 1998;6:36–43
7. Shah SA. Scheuermann kyphosis. In: Albert TJ, Heary RF, ed. Spinal Deformity: The Essentials, Vol 1. New York: Thieme; 2014:163–174
8. Dimar JR II, Glassman SD, Carreon LY. Juvenile degenerative disc disease: a report of 76 cases identified by magnetic resonance imaging. Spine J 2007;7:332–337
9. Ogilvie JW, Sherman J. Spondylolysis in Scheuermann's disease. Spine 1987;12:251–253
10. Lonner B, Yoo A, Terran JS, et al. Effect of spinal deformity on adolescent quality of life: comparison of operative Scheuermann kyphosis, adolescent idiopathic scoliosis, and normal controls. Spine 2013;38:1049–1055
11. Ristolainen L, Kettunen JA, Heliövaara M, Kujala UM, Heinonen A, Schlenzka D. Untreated Scheuermann's disease: a 37-year follow-up study. Eur Spine J 2012;21:819–824
12. Othman Z, Lenke LG, Bolon SM, Padberg A. Hypotension-induced loss of intraoperative monitoring data during surgical correction of Scheuermann kyphosis: a case report. Spine 2004;29:E258–E265
13. Gutman G, Labelle H, Barchi S, Roussouly P, Berthonnaud É, Mac-Thiong JM. Normal sagittal parameters of global spinal balance in children and adolescents: a prospective study of 646 asymptomatic subjects. Eur Spine J 2016;25:3650–3657
14. Fisk JW, Baigent ML, Hill PD. Scheuermann's disease. Clinical and radiological survey of 17 and 18 year olds. Am J Phys Med 1984;63:18–30
15. Lowe TG. Scheuermann Disease. Philadelphia: Lippincott-Raven; 1997

16. Bradford DS, Moe JH, Montalvo FJ, Winter RB. Scheuermann's kyphosis and roundback deformity. Results of Milwaukee brace treatment. J Bone Joint Surg Am 1974;56:740–758

17. Gutowski WT, Renshaw TS. Orthotic results in adolescent kyphosis. Spine 1988;13:485–489

18. Sturm PF, Dobson JC, Armstrong GW. The surgical management of Scheuermann's disease. Spine 1993; 18:685–691

19. Smith-Petersen MN, Larson CB, Aufranc OE. Osteotomy of the spine for correction of flexion deformity in rheumatoid arthritis. Clin Orthop Relat Res 1969; 66:6–9

20. Geck MJ, Macagno A, Ponte A, Shufflebarger HL. The Ponte procedure: posterior only treatment of Scheuermann's kyphosis using segmental posterior shortening and pedicle screw instrumentation. J Spinal Disord Tech 2007;20:586–593

21. Lonner BS, Newton P, Betz R, et al. Operative management of Scheuermann's kyphosis in 78 patients: radiographic outcomes, complications, and technique. Spine 2007;32:2644–2652

22. Lowe TG, Kasten MD. An analysis of sagittal curves and balance after Cotrel-Dubousset instrumentation for kyphosis secondary to Scheuermann's disease. A review of 32 patients. Spine 1994;19:1680–1685

23. Denis F, Sun EC, Winter RB. Incidence and risk factors for proximal and distal junctional kyphosis following surgical treatment for Scheuermann kyphosis: minimum five-year follow-up. Spine 2009;34:E729–E734

24. Boachie-Adjei O, Bradford DS. Vertebral column resection and arthrodesis for complex spinal deformities. J Spinal Disord 1991;4:193–202

25. Deviren V, Scheer JK, Ames CP. Technique of cervicothoracic junction pedicle subtraction osteotomy for cervical sagittal imbalance: report of 11 cases. J Neurosurg Spine 2011;15:174–181

26. Poolman RW, Been HD, Ubags LH. Clinical outcome and radiographic results after operative treatment of Scheuermann's disease. Eur Spine J 2002;11:561–569

27. Cho KJ, Lenke LG, Bridwell KH, Kamiya M, Sides B. Selection of the optimal distal fusion level in posterior instrumentation and fusion for thoracic hyperkyphosis: the sagittal stable vertebra concept. Spine 2009;34:765–770

28. Nasto LA, Perez-Romera AB, Shalabi ST, Quraishi NA, Mehdian H. Correlation between preoperative spino-pelvic alignment and risk of proximal junctional kyphosis after posterior-only surgical correction of Scheuermann kyphosis. Spine J 2016;16(4, Suppl): S26–S33

29. Lonner BS, Toombs CS, Guss M, et al. Complications in operative Scheuermann kyphosis: do the pitfalls differ from operative adolescent idiopathic scoliosis? Spine 2015;40:305–311

30. Ain MC, Shirley ED. Spinal fusion for kyphosis in achondroplasia. J Pediatr Orthop 2004;24:541–545

31. Misra SN, Morgan HW. Thoracolumbar spinal deformity in achondroplasia. Neurosurg Focus 2003;14:e4

32. Winter RB, Moe JH, Wang JF. Congenital kyphosis. Its natural history and treatment as observed in a study of one hundred and thirty patients. J Bone Joint Surg Am 1973;55:223–256

33. Zeller RD, Ghanem I, Dubousset J. The congenital dislocated spine. Spine 1996;21:1235–1240

34. Mayfield JK, Winter RB, Bradford DS, Moe JH. Congenital kyphosis due to defects of anterior segmentation. J Bone Joint Surg Am 1980;62:1291–1301

35. Kim YJ, Otsuka NY, Flynn JM, Hall JE, Emans JB, Hresko MT. Surgical treatment of congenital kyphosis. Spine 2001;26:2251–2257

36. Ginsburg GM, Lauder AJ. Progression of scoliosis in patients with spastic quadriplegia after the insertion of an intrathecal baclofen pump. Spine 2007;32: 2745–2750

37. Vialle R, Thévenin-Lemoine C, Mary P. Neuromuscular scoliosis. Orthop Traumatol Surg Res 2013;99(1, Suppl):S124–S139

38. Dayer R, Ouellet JA, Saran N. Pelvic fixation for neuromuscular scoliosis deformity correction. Curr Rev Musculoskelet Med 2012;5:91–101

39. Askin GN, Hallett R, Hare N, Webb JK. The outcome of scoliosis surgery in the severely physically handicapped child. An objective and subjective assessment. Spine 1997;22:44–50

40. Tsuchiya K, Bridwell KH, Kuklo TR, Lenke LG, Baldus C. Minimum 5-year analysis of L5-S1 fusion using sacropelvic fixation (bilateral S1 and iliac screws) for spinal deformity. Spine 2006;31:303–308

41. Amhaz HH, Fox BD, Johnson KK, et al. Postlaminoplasty kyphotic deformity in the thoracic spine: case report and review of the literature. Pediatr Neurosurg 2009;45:151–154

15

Spine Surgery in the Developing World

Oheneba Boachie-Adjei and Irene Adorkor Wulff

⠿ Introduction

The United Nations has classified countries on the basis of their state of economic and social development as least developed, developing, transitional, and developed; 48 countries are considered least developed, 95 developing, 22 transitional, and 26 developed.[1,2] Musculoskeletal diseases continue to produce major disability around the world.[3,4] Approximately half of the world's population has no access to orthopedic care, including pediatric spine deformity care, which is a highly specialized area of orthopedic care. The problem is made worse by the lack of qualified personnel, the inadequate facilities, and the inability of patients to access the few existing facilities.[5] The combination of these factors has led many patients to live with severe and neglected spine deformities. The relative distribution of causes of death differs markedly between developed and developing countries. Of special interest to orthopedic surgeons is the prominence of tuberculosis, the sequelae of motor vehicle accidents, and congenital anomalies as causes of death in developing nations.[4–6] Spine surgery has benefited from the extraordinary developments of spine assessment, imaging, and complex surgical techniques of instrumentation in recent decades. These benefits are lacking in the developing world because even basic radiographic studies for spine deformity assessment are often nonexistent.[5,7]

Families of pediatric patients with spine deformities often lack the financial resources to seek medical care, and thus they turn to alternative and ineffective treatments. These patients present a unique challenge in developing nations such as Ghana, where there is not a single trained spine deformity surgeon for 26 million people.[8] Those who are fortunate enough to obtain surgical treatment after failed conservative methods present with a myriad of medical comorbidities and advanced deformities, and thus they pose significant challenges to the medical treatment team. A multidisciplinary approach is needed to manage these patients perioperatively for successful outcomes. Patients presenting to our institution in Ghana are managed with a variety of nonsurgical and surgical methods customized to suit patients' deformities and the available long-term care. A significant number of pediatric patients with complex spine deformities with restrictive pulmonary disease have to be managed with long-term preoperative halo gravity traction, a nutritional optimization program, and complex surgical interventions and postoperative management for successful outcomes.[9,10]

The best way to circumvent the obstacles associated with the management of pediatric spine deformities is for their early detection and treatment to be among the leading major health concerns in the minds, actions, and funding priorities of international health agencies, governments, nongovernmental organizations, funders, and the general public.[5,11] We have embraced this mission of the Bone and Joint Decade at the Foundation of *Orthopaedics* and Complex Spine (FOCOS) Orthopaedic Hospital in Ghana, and we hope to facilitate establishing an infrastructure for sustainable programs and services in the West Africa subregion. Due to the complexity of spine deformities and the lack of resources, a good way to establish a treatment center is to follow the guidelines developed by the Scoliosis Research Society.

Spine Deformity and Disorders in the Developing World

All manner of spine deformities and disorders are seen in the developing world. At our center in Ghana, the majority of patients present with scoliosis, which is the most common pediatric deformity. It is idiopathic in origin in 75 to 90% of cases (**Fig. 15.1**). The remaining 10 to 25% may be secondary to congenital anomalies,

neuromuscular disease, infection, tumor, injury, or as part of such syndromes as Marfan's and neurofibromatosis. Of utmost importance is that many patients present with severe early-onset spine deformity and failure to thrive. Casting or bracing facilities are not available in many underserved regions for these patients, leaving surgery as the only treatment option available.

For adolescent patients who have gone untreated, the deformities most often exceed 100 degrees in one or two planes and are associated with severe restrictive lung disease. A forced vital capacity (FVC) below 40% is a common presentation. We have assessed the nutritional state of our pediatric population and have recognized that 90% of these patients were undernourished or small for their age.[12] Using height to determine the patient's body mass index (BMI) is very misleading, so we have resorted to using the arm span as a proxy for height in calculating an appropriate and meaningful BMI. Moreover, one cannot always use the chronological age as a factor in deciding on the surgical treatment of patients with early-onset scoliosis, as is done in developed countries;

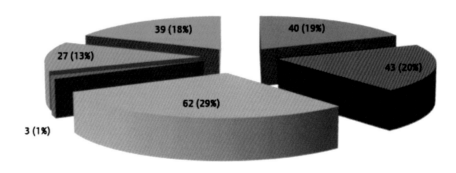

- Scoliosis
- Kyphosis
- Kyphoscoliosis
- Cervical stenosis and prolapse
- Lumbar stenosis and disc prolapse
- Others (syrinx, tumor, staged procedures, revisions, incision and drainage)

Fig. 15.1 Number of patients (and percents) in the diagnostic categories of the spine deformity cases seen during 1 year at the FOCOS Hospital.

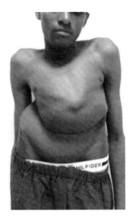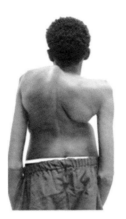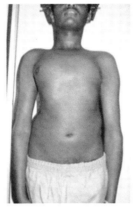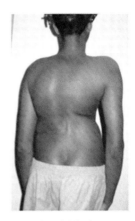

b

Fig. 15.2 Preoperative and 5 months postoperative halo traction with aggressive nutritional intervention in an adolescent boy with kyphoscoliosis. **(a)** Preoperative front and back view. **(b)** After 5 months of nutritional optimization and halo gravity traction (HGT). The preoperative pulmonary function test (PFT) demonstrated restrictive lung disease with forced vital capacity (FVC) (L) of 1.15 (29%); forced expiratory volume in 1 second (FEV_1) (L) of 0.98 (28%); and FEV_1/FVC (%) of 84.9 (103%). After 5 months of traction, the PFT was as follows: FVC (L), 1.87 (45%); FEV_1 (L), 1.62 (45%); FEV_1/FVC (%), 88 (102%).

instead, we use skeletal age, and have instituted growing rod treatment programs in some 12- and 13-year-olds who present with skeletal age 6 or 7. Growing rod or growth friendly treatment includes utilization of limited fusion of the spine, allowing the unfused spine to grow. Periodic lengthenings are done to keep up with longitudinal growth of the spine. Early identification of patients who are malnourished or at risk is essential to institute timely nutrition interventions. Our nutritional optimization program has achieved improvements in weight and BMI prior to surgical intervention in a significant number of patients (**Fig. 15.2**).

Tuberculosis (TB) spondylitis leading to post-TB kyphosis is prevalent in the developing world and causes some of the most severe kyphotic deformities and paralysis. It is not uncommon to see very young patients presenting with severe kyphosis exceeding 100 degrees, with neurologic impairment.[9,13] Medical management is still the mainstay of nonoperative treatment and is available through public health programs in most developing countries.[14] Surgical intervention is reserved for those with radiographic at-risk signs as described by Rajasekaran and associates.[15] Patients with neurologic deficits, severe and painful deformities, or pulmonary compromise are considered candidates for surgical intervention.

Clinical Presentation

Our pediatric patients range in age from 12 months to 21 years, and they hail from different countries in Africa. They usually are not accompanied by a parent at the time of presentation for surgical treatment. The parents and guardians of some of the patients have been met during outreach visitations to the countries of origin by members of the FOCOS team, who have had the opportunity to discuss treatment options with them and their referring physicians. This sometimes presents an ethical dilemma when it comes to obtaining informed consent for complex spine surgery. The senior author and referring physicians communicate all treatment plans and complications with the families or guardians for a comprehensive consent before the patients depart for treatment in Ghana. Out-of-state patients are accompanied by a caregiver who also serves as the interpreter and proxy guardian to provide additional treatment consents.

Upon presentation to the clinic, a comprehensive assessment is done, which includes a medical, physical, and spinal exam. An angle of trunk rotation (ATR) exceeding 30 degrees, which falls outside the limits of the scoliometer device, is very common. A thorough neurologic evaluation is performed and documented using the American Spinal Injury Association (ASIA) grading system. Older children are given the English version of the Scoliosis Research Society Outcomes Questionnaire (SRS-22), a health-related quality-of-life (HRQOL) instrument, to complete.[16] We have recently compared the preoperative SRS-22 results of patients from Ghana, patients from New York City, and controls who were matched for age and sex. Adolescents without scoliosis had significantly better scores than scoliotic adolescents. Ghanaian scoliotic adolescents had significantly worse HRQOL scores than American scoliotic adolescents. These differences should be kept in mind when treating the emotionally vulnerable adolescent population in developing nations.

Radiographic studies including standard standing or upright anteroposterior and lateral views on 36-inch-long films are obtained to evaluate curve magnitude, type, and etiology. Many developing countries lack sophisticated radiographic imaging facilities and have to rely on radiographs not depicting the entire spine on a single film. In such cases, practitioners must piece together segments of the radiographic images to assess curve magnitude and etiology. Several radiographs may be needed to evaluate specific segments of the spine, resulting in increased radiation exposure and cost.

Patients with curves exceeding 100 degrees in either plane with less than 20% flexibility are considered candidates for a halo gravity traction program.[10] Advanced imaging is very hard to come by in many developing countries, and one may have to rely on only a careful review of the plain radiographs and a detailed neurologic assessment to make treatment decisions. Access is also limited. Ghana, for example, currently has 10 magnetic resonance imaging (MRI) and 20 computed tomography (CT) scan machines for 26 million people. The cost may also be prohibitive for many patients. We strive to obtain an MRI on all neurologically impaired

patients and those with congenital anomalies preoperatively. For the latter group of patients, an echocardiogram and renal ultrasound is also obtained, as these patients have been found to have a higher incidence of associated anomalies of these organ systems[17] At our center, a global fee scale has been developed for surgical patients who are able to afford the nominal charges, which includes all treatment modalities, professional fees, imaging, hospital stay, and laboratory studies.

Medical and Anesthetic Considerations

Even though a multidisciplinary approach is preferred to manage spine deformity patients, such specialists may not be available in underserved regions. Thus, the preoperative evaluation should determine the presence of associated medical conditions and should try to obtain the records of previous medical and surgical procedures. Common coexisting medical conditions encountered in the West Africa subregion include tuberculosis, sickle cell disease, viral hepatitis, and HIV. Patient with these conditions or high viral titers are counseled to postpone surgical intervention and consider medical management accordingly.

The etiology, location, and degree of the deformity should be noted, and any other congenital abnormalities should be investigated to plan the most appropriate procedure for the particular case. This will enable a meaningful estimation of the duration and complexity of surgery, and preparation for potential complications. Particular attention should be paid to the respiratory and cardiovascular systems as well as to the central nervous system (CNS). Patients with severe spine deformities may have wheezes on chest examination. The presence of dyspnea at rest or on minimal exertion, orthopnea, or paroxysmal nocturnal dyspnea is indicative of imminent cardiac failure and loss of cardiovascular reserve. These conditions are occasionally seen in very severe deformities exceeding 100 degrees in young patients. Included in our risk stratification protocol are

Table 15.1 FOCOS Level Score Sheet of Patient Shown in Fig. 15.2a, with Level 5 High-Risk Score Downgraded to Level 4 Postoperatively

Category	Points (Preoperative)	Points (Post-Traction)	Points (Postoperative)	Maximum Points Allowed
Maximum deformity	40	40	40	40
American Society of Anesthesiologists (ASA)	6	6	6	10
Body mass index (BMI)	8	6	6	10
American Spinal Injury Association (ASIA) score	2	2	2	10
Fusion levels	8	8	8	10
Osteotomy	20	20	5	20
Total	84	82	71	100
Risk score	5A	5A	4B	
Level grade	Very high	Very high	Moderately high	

the American Society of Anesthesiologists (ASA) measurement, the BMI, the etiology, the curve magnitude, the Fusion levels, the osteotomy type, and the neurologic status. An electrocardiogram (ECG), a pulmonary function test (PFT), and echocardiography, if available, should be ordered preoperatively. Cervical mobility and upper airway anatomy are also assessed to determine any potential airway or positioning difficulties (**Table 15.1**).

Preparation should be made for the possibility of blood transfusion, for prolonged stay in the intensive care unit (ICU), and for postoperative pain management. These modalities are discussed with the patient and guardian as part of the informed consent interview.

Respiratory Effects and Postoperative Considerations

The FVC is a reliable prognostic indicator of perioperative respiratory reserve.[18] Based on our knowledge that patients with severe curves or neuromuscular disease have poor pulmonary function and may have a stormy postoperative course, we routinely ventilate patients postoperatively for 12 to 24 hours. This has reduced reintubation events in the middle of the night when resources and staff are limited. We highly recommend such protocols when treating severe spine deformity patients in developing countries (**Fig. 15.2**).

Cardiovascular Function

Congenital spine deformity may also be associated with congenital heart conditions such as mitral valve prolapse, coarctation, cyanotic heart disease, and congenital chest wall abnormalities leading to thoracic insufficiency syndrome. Pulmonary hypertension may result in right-heart failure and eventually death.

Anesthetic Techniques

Important anesthetic considerations in surgery for spinal deformity include management of the patient in the prone position, hypothermia secondary to a long procedure with an extensive exposed area, replacement of blood and fluid losses that may be extensive, maintenance of spinal cord integrity, and blood conservation techniques. A general anesthetic technique with intubation and mechanical ventilation is used in pediatric spine deformity surgery in all regions of the world.[19] The aim is to maintain an adequate depth of anesthesia, which enables intraoperative neurophysiological monitoring, if available. Our protocol includes hemodynamic monitoring, preoxygenation, intravenous induction with midazolam 0.1 mg/kg, fentanyl 5 µg/kg, and propofol 150 to 300 mg. This enables tracheal intubation without the use of a muscle relaxant. Bite blocks are inserted to prevent the tongue bites during stimulation of motor evoked potentials (MEPs). Maintenance of anesthesia is done with propofol, fentanyl, and oxygen.

Routine hemodynamic monitoring intraoperatively includes invasive blood pressure (BP) assessment via a radial artery cannula. BP measurement starts at induction in patients with cardiac instability. A central line is not always available, and therefore it is not routinely used intraoperatively. We have performed hundreds of complex spine procedures in pediatric patients without the central line, with very favorable outcomes. The central line is only placed when there is significant morbidity or difficult peripheral intravenous access. A urethral catheter is inserted routinely to monitor urine output and hence tissue perfusion.

Intraoperative Considerations

The prone patient positioning requires good, coordinated teamwork as accidental extubation or dislodgment of intravascular and urinary catheters can occur. Blindness, though rare, has been reported after spine surgery, and has been attributed to multiple causes such as anemia, hypotension, and improper positioning.[20] The padding of the eyes is therefore frequently checked during surgery. Vulnerable areas such as peripheral nerves and genitalia should be protected from compression and soft tissue damage. The arms are anteriorly flexed and abducted to reduce tension on the brachial plexus. Invasive BP monitoring is started at this point, and noninvasive BP monitoring is set at 30-minute intervals for intermittent comparison.

Surgical Planning, Preparation, and Intervention

Surgical treatment of pediatric patients in developing countries is fraught with potential problems. The deformities are severe and neglected. The patients present with a myriad of comorbidities that were addressed above. When a patient is finally considered to be a candidate for surgical intervention, we determine the surgical risk score based on several risk factors. We have recently published a new method for surgical risk stratification.[12] The risk level is classified from 1 (low risk) to 5 (high risk). In our system at FOCOS, we determine the risk level based on the scores on our stratification questionnaire, as follow: level 1, 1 to 20 points; level 2, 21 to 40 points; level 3, 41 to 60 points; level 4, 61 to 80 points); and level 5, 81 to 100 points. Multiple regression analysis indicated a significant correlation between FOCOS level and estimated blood loss, length of surgery, and neurologic and overall complication ratio (**Table 15.2**). This assessment has allowed us to carefully select and prepare pediatric patients for complex spine surgical intervention. Severe and stiff deformities with restrictive pulmonary disease are considered for long-term halo gravity traction (HGT). Our halo gravity protocol includes starting at 20% body weight and increasing it by 10% per week until 50% body weight is achieved. In our review of patients treated with this method, scoliosis improved from an average of 131 degrees to

Table 15.2 FOCOS Risk Score and Complication Rate

FOCOS Level	Number of Patients	Percent of Neuro-monitoring Change (N)	Percent of Complications (N)	Percent of Neurologic Complications (N)	% of Estimated Blood Loss/ Total Blood Volume	Time of Surgery (Minutes)
1	5	0 (0)	0 (0)	0 (0)	26.9 ± 19.5	240.8 ± 84.8
2	19	15.8 (3)	5.3 (1)	0 (0)	32.9 ± 5.3	267.5 ± 97.1
3	25	16.0 (4)	32.0 (8)	0 (0)	53.4 ± 39.8	318.6 ± 109.6
4	58	39.7 (23)	41.4 (24)	5.2 (3)	50.4 ± 27.3	348.2 ± 135.1
5	38	42.1 (16)	31.6 (12)	10.5 (4)	56.6 ± 24.2	367.2 ± 169.1

91 degrees (31%). Pure kyphotics improved an average of 22%. Deformity correction with HGT plateaued at 63 days. There were no neurologic complications. We were able to demonstrate that long-term HGT is safe and provides curve correction as well as improves the pulmonary function, and in most cases has obviated the need for complex and high-risk three-column osteotomies, especially when resources are limited. For patients with early-onset spine deformities with severe kyphoscoliosis, the HGT has been shown to significantly improve the curves to render them amenable to growth-friendly instrumentation (**Figs. 15.2** and **15.3**).

The spinal cord is at risk of injury during corrective spine surgery and when the spinal canal is surgically invaded, such as in three-column osteotomy procedures. The incidence of motor deficit or paraplegia after surgery to correct scoliosis in the absence of spinal cord monitoring techniques has been quoted as between 3.7% and 6.9%.[10,14,21] This has been reduced by intraoperative monitoring (IOM) to 0.5%. In the developed world, spinal cord monitoring is a standard practice and plays a major role in the management of complex pediatric deformities.[9,13,21] This modality is not available in many treatment centers in the developing world, so the surgical team has to resort to the wake-up test. This may take some time because advanced anesthetic methods for total intravenous anesthesia (TIVA) with medications like remifentanil may not be available. Patience is therefore required during the reversal process of waking up the patient. When dealing with patients who speak a language different from the that of the surgical team, a preoperative rehearsal of the wake-up test with an interpreter is crucial.

⫶ Intraoperative Blood Loss

It is well known that spine deformity surgery can result in excessive blood loss, which may, in some cases, exceed circulating blood volume. Factors influencing the degree of blood loss include the number of levels fused, the duration of surgery, and the presence of hypother-

mia. At our center, very young patients present with severe deformities along with low BMI and hence low total blood volume. It is therefore very common to reach a high percentage of the total blood volume loss in these small patients within a short operative period. In developing countries there is immense pressure on the limited blood inventory. Homologous blood transfusion is also associated with the risks of transmission of bacterial and viral infections, alloimmunization, immunomodulation, graft versus host disease, metabolic imbalance, and transfusion mismatch. These potential risks necessitate the institution of measures to minimize homologous blood transfusion. It is important to monitor volume status and blood loss carefully in these patients, with regular hemoglobin, platelet, and coagulation estimations. A portable hand-held device like the HemoCue is perfect for these settings with limited resources.

Blood Conservation Methods

Correct patient positioning to reduce intra-abdominal pressure minimizes epidural venous engorgement and venous surgical bleeding. It is imperative to execute good aseptic surgical technique and hemostasis, and to minimize soft tissue damage.

Hypotensive anesthesia (reduction of systolic pressure 20 mm Hg from baseline or lowering mean arterial pressure to 65 mm Hg) in the normotensive patient has been shown to decrease blood loss, reduce transfusion requirements by 50%, and shorten operating times.[22,23] Various agents can be used to achieve this, including nitroglycerine, α- and β-blockers, ganglion blocking drugs such as trimethaphan and sodium nitroprusside, calcium channel blockers such as nicardipine, volatile anaesthetics, and fenoldopam. Although these agents are desirable, they may not be available in most developing countries. Labetalol and nitroglycerine are used in our institution.

Antifibrinolytic agents such as tranexamic acid competitively inhibits activation of plasminogen, thereby reducing conversion of plasminogen to plasmin, an enzyme that degrades

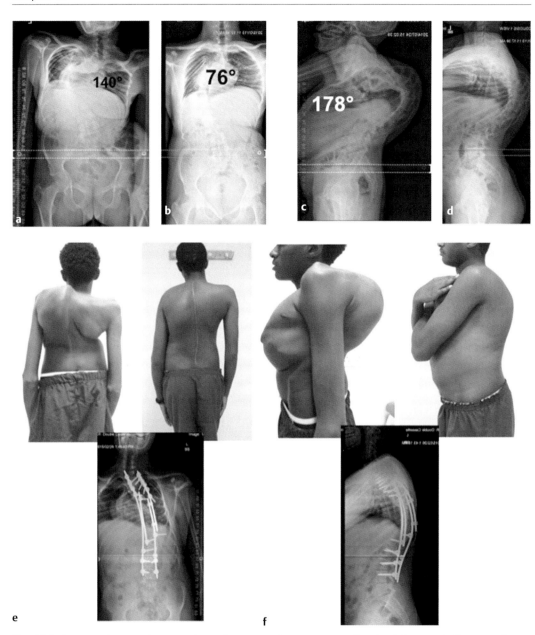

Fig. 15.3 Preoperative anterior posterior radiographs of the adolescent boy shown in **Fig. 15.2**. **(a)** The coronal curve measures 140 degrees. **(b)** After 5 months of HGT, scoliosis improves to 76 degrees. **(c)** Preoperative lateral view shows severe kyphosis of 178 degrees. **(d)** After 5 months of HGT, improvement of kyphosis is seen. **(e,f)** Pre- and postoperative clinical photos and radiographs after one-stage posterior spine fusion instrumentation, posterior column osteotomies, and rib resections. Note the clinical and radiographic improvement.

fibrin clots. Tranexamic acid also directly inhibits plasmin activity at higher dosages.[24] In our institution, tranexamic acid is infused throughout surgery at 10 mg/kg/h for the first hour and at 1 mg/kg/h thereafter.

Autologous Blood

The use of autologous blood can also reduce the need for allogenic transfusions. This may be done by pre-donation, intraoperative acute normovolemic hemodilution, or intraoperative cell salvage.[22] This facility may be difficult to implement in most developing countries. Several weeks prior to surgery, basic laboratory bloodwork is obtained, and patients with low hemoglobin are placed on oral iron supplementation to minimize preoperative anemia. We do not routinely practice autologous predonation or use recombinant erythropoietin due to the costs associated with these modalities.

Acute Normovolemic Hemodilution

Acute normovolemic hemodilution (ANH) is the removal, soon after anesthetic induction, of a predetermined volume of blood, which is reinfused during or preferably at completion of the procedure.[22] Normovolemia is maintained by the simultaneous replacement with crystalloids or colloids. The rationale is that during the ensuing surgery, the patient will lose blood of low hematocrit. Fresh blood is thus available at the end of surgery and is beneficial should a coagulopathy occur. Patients selected for ANH should have hemoglobin of ≥ 12 g/dL and should have no significant cardiovascular, renal, or cerebral insufficiency. A recent review of matched cohorts of ANH and non-ANH patients at out institution showed that ANH can be safely performed in complex spine surgery in underserved geographic regions. The ANH patients received lower volume allogenic blood transfusion to attain the same postoperative hemoglobin levels.

Intraoperative Blood Salvage

Intraoperative blood salvage (IBS) has been found to significantly reduce the use of homol-ogous red blood cells (RBCs).[25] Again, this technique may be unavailable in most developing countries due to costs and to the lack of equipment and personnel. We have employed IBS at our institution when the blood loss is expected to be more than 20% of the total circulating blood volume of the patient. ANH and IBS are the main sources of autologous blood at our institution.

Intraoperative Neuromonitoring

The anesthetic technique can have profound effects on the ability to monitor spinal cord function. There are three main methods of IOM used in our institution: the Stagnara wake-up test, somatosensory evoked potentials (SSEPs), and MEPs. During the wake-up test, all anesthetic agents are turned off, opioids are reversed, any neuromuscular blockade is reversed, and the patient is allowed to wake up and is asked to move his or her hands and feet. Once shown to be intact, the patient is again anesthetized to allow completion of the procedure. The wake-up test assesses spinal cord function only at that one specific time and not continuously during the procedure. We perform the wake-up test in patients with very severe deformities when the MEPs are lost and all other factors such as hypotension, hypothermia, hypercarbia, and interference by anesthetic agents are ruled out. False negatives occur sometimes. Because advance modalities such as transcranial MEP and SSEP are not available in most underserved regions, we advise the surgical team to be very conversant with the wake-up test.

Surgical Techniques

A variety of surgical approaches are available for treating pediatric spine deformities. They include posterior spinal fusion with or without instrumentation, anterior spine fusion with or without instrumentation, and combined anterior and posterior procedures. The use of segmental instrumentation such as pedicle screws has reduced the incidence of performing combined procedures due to the inherent power of the pedicle screws to correct spine deformity, especially when combined with osteotomy techniques. C-arm fluoroscopy is rarely available in most operating rooms in developing countries. It is therefore imperative that surgeons master the technique of free-hand pedicle screw placement. A careful review of the preoperative radiographs to assess pedicle dimension and anatomy will aid in safe screw placement. When there is difficulty in placing screws with this method, a small laminotomy to feel the medial pedicle wall with a Penfield dissector helps with screw placement and trajectory.

Posterior Approaches

The most commonly used surgical approach is posterior segmental instrumentation and fusion with or without posterior column osteotomies. It is a simpler and more familiar approach, performed in a single stage, with less operative time and blood loss. For FOCOS level 1 to 3 deformities, a good outcome can be expected with the posterior-only approach. Posterior segmental instrumentation with hybrid or all-pedicle-screw constructs will suffice for these level 1 to 3 deformities. We try to reduce the implant density to an average of 60 to 80% by selecting strategic levels for implant fixation to achieve optimal and balanced correction in all planes. We have not found any negative outcomes from such practice (**Fig. 15.4**). For patients with severe and rigid curves who have been in preoperative traction, the surgical procedure is performed in traction utilizing 50% of the preoperative traction weights divided equally between the head and both feet. In such cases we will also resort to performing concave rib osteotomies, convex thoracoplasties, and Ponte osteotomies to achieve safe curve correction without a three-column osteotomy. Patients with FVC > 30% who have a non-neuromuscular condition are able to tolerate this treatment method and can be successfully extubated without the need for tracheotomy. Patients with sharp angular deformities are best treated with posterior three-column osteotomies. Most are managed in a one-stage fashion, especially for hyperkyphotic deformities[26,27] (**Fig. 15.5**). However, if the surgery is running long and the patient has lost > 50% of the blood volume prior to the resection portion of the procedure, or is neurologically or pulmonary unstable, we stage the procedure and place a temporary rod. The second stage is usually performed a week or two later when

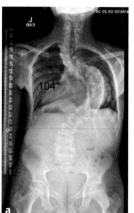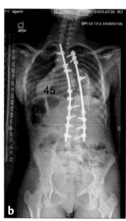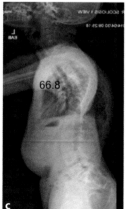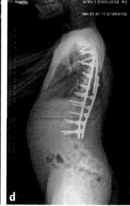

Fig. 15.4 Pre- and postoperative radiographs of a 14-year-old girl with adolescent idiopathic scoliosis (AIS) and FOCOS level 3 treated with posterior spine fusion, temporary internal distraction, segmental instrumentation, and thoracoplasty. **(a,b)** Pre- and postoperative anteroposterior (AP) views. **(c,d)** Postoperative lateral views.

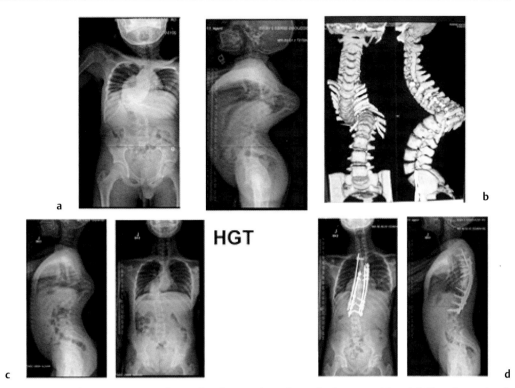

Fig. 15.5 Pre- and postoperative radiographs of a 16-year-old boy with complex vertebral transposition (gamma deformity) treated with 6 months of HGT and vertebral column resection. **(a)** Preoperative AP and lateral radiographs. **(b)** Preoperative computed tomography (CT) scans show coronal and lateral vertebral transposition. **(c)** After 6 months of HGT, there is improvement of transposition in both planes. **(d)** Postoperative AP and lateral radiographs show spinal realignment in the coronal and sagittal planes.

the patient is hemodynamically and neurologically stable.

Combined Anterior and Posterior Approaches

Combined anterior and posterior procedures are less commonly performed in many centers nowadays due to their associated morbidity and their effect on the already compromised pulmonary function of severely deformed pediatric patients. Treatment centers in developing countries may not have access to surgeons for the anterior approach or the resources to manage these patients postoperatively, which requires intensive care unit facilities and equipment such as chest tubes. Moreover, the use of posterior segmental fixation with pedicle screws coupled with posterior three-column osteotomies have allowed effective correction of deformities without the anterior release and fusion. There are instances, however, where anterior surgery is needed to prevent the crankshaft phenomenon in very immature patients and in patients for whom anterior column support is needed to fill a void after a posterior procedure. This is performed in ~ 10% of the patients presenting to our institution. Infections with epidural abscesses and cord compression will require anterior debridement and decompression. During the vertebral column resection procedure, the anterior column is reconstructed with bone or titanium mesh cage. Failure to achieve adequate anterior column load sharing will be an indication for a supplemental anterior approach.

Growth-Friendly Surgical Techniques

Young children with spinal deformities are at the highest risk of suffering permanent pulmonary impairment with an eventual decrease in life expectancy.[28] Children with progressive early-onset scoliosis may benefit from early operative treatment with dual growing rods, which provide an "internal brace" for the spine and allow curve correction and sequential lengthening to maximize thoracic cage development.[29–31] Unfortunately, in developing countries patients with early-onset scoliosis seek medical attention very late and have severe deformities that make placing a growing rod very challenging. Serial casting or bracing is virtually nonexistent in many developing countries. There are few orthopedic cast technicians and few cast and bracing materials available to manage early-onset scoliosis patients. On the other hand, few facilities can afford the luxury of performing repeated operations and managing the complications associated with repeated surgeries.[29,30] Follow-up is also a big problem in that patients may come from long distances and cannot afford the cost associated with the long-term treatment. Spinal instrumentation for pediatric patients is also not readily available in most developing countries.

Fraught with these problems, we have sought to treat these patients with low-cost and modified instrumentation constructs. For those with mild or moderate and flexible curves, we have performed a modified growth-guided procedure to enable the instrumentation to lengthen with the natural growth of the spine. We have called this technique the FOCOS bidirectional growth modulation (FBGM) (**Fig. 15.6**). Our current indications include patients with skeletal age less than 8 years for boys and 6 years for girls, with curves up to 70 degrees and with 50% flexibility. Several patients meeting these criteria have been successfully treated and are under periodic observation. Older patients with larger curves are treated with a standard dual-rod distraction system and are followed with an 8- to 12-month lengthening program.

For severe and rigid early-onset scoliotic deformities > 100 degrees, we have instituted the long-term HGT method for an average of 62 days to improve curve flexibility prior to instituting a growing rod treatment program. The traction techniques provide ~ 30% correction and also aid in nutrition and pulmonary function optimization. Despite not having casting facilities in underserved regions, the deformities are too severe to warrant cast application. Standard distraction growing rod instrumentation is kyphogenic and is relatively

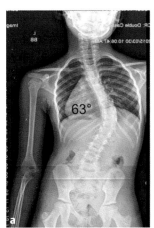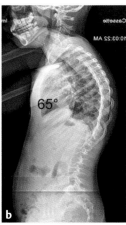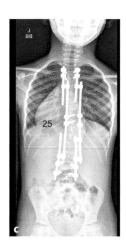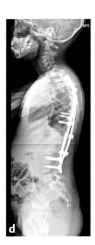

Fig. 15.6 Pre- and postoperative radiographs of a 6-year-old girl with idiopathic early-onset scoliosis treated with the FOCOS bidirectional growth modulation (FBGM) technique. **(a,b)** Preoperative AP and lateral radiographs. **(c,d)** Postoperative AP and lateral radiographs showing multiple-rod fixation with end fusion and apical fusion and sliding periapical connectors and rods.

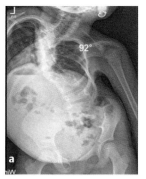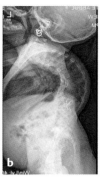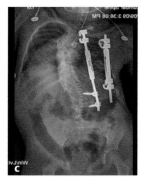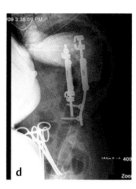

Fig. 15.7 Pre- and postoperative radiographs of a 7-year-old girl with congenital scoliosis and rib cage deformities treated with thoracoplasties and modified vertebral expandable prosthetic titanium ribs (VEPTRs). **(a,b)** Preoperative AP and lateral radiographs. **(c,d)** Postoperative AP and lateral radiographs show proximal hook claws at T2-T3 and distal pedicle screws at L2–L3.

contraindicated in patients starting out with severe kyphosis. For such patients the long-term halo gravity method has significantly reduced the preoperative hyperkyphosis, making them amenable to successful growing rod distraction instrumentation. Another common complication of distraction systems is proximal junctional kyphosis. For this reason we have routinely instrumented proximally to T1 or T2 and in some case up to C7.

In developed countries, patients with congenital and chest wall deformities may be treated with rib and chest wall expansion devices or magnetically driven distraction instrumentation. In Ghana, a modified chest wall distraction instrumentation made up of standard hooks and rods is utilized. Several types of construct combinations, such as rib to rib and rib to spine, are considered based on the type of deformity (**Fig. 15.7**).

Three-Column Osteotomies

Pedicle subtraction osteotomy (PSO) and vertebral column resection (VCR) are the most complicated of the three-column osteotomies, and they pose a substantial neurologic risk to the patient.[21,31,32] But they are indicated for sharp angular kyphosis and for severe and rigid multiplanar deformities.[33] These procedures are indicated for the type of complex and untreated deformities that are found in developing countries where resources are also limited. Other instances where the posterior vertebral column resection is the only viable surgical option include congenital, posttraumatic, and postinfectious kyphosis > 100 degrees.[15,28]

Surgical Technique

The hallmark of the VCR procedure is posterior circumspinal resection, posterior shortening, and anterior column lengthening.[31,33,34] A recent study from our center has reported that the risk of neurologic injury is highest when the apex is thoracic, between T6 and T10.[26] We would therefore suggest that surgeons undertaking the posterior VCR procedure in the mid-thoracic segment of the spine exercise caution. A case in point are deformities that we have characterized as omega and gamma in that the curve magnitudes exceed 180 degrees in one or two planes (**Fig. 15.2**). For these deformities, we have utilized long-term HGT to unwind the spine and "uncross" the transposed apical segments as well as improve the periapical segment compensatory deformities. We postulate that HGT enables gradual stretching to "train" the cord to tolerate the definitive surgical procedure that adds another 20 to 30% correction without rapidly applying undue force to achieve the maximum. The VCR procedure requires technical expertise, intraoperative neuromonitoring, and the blood salvage methods described above, all of which we have been able to establish at our institution.

Postoperative Medical Management

Most pediatric spine deformity patients are extubated immediately after surgery to enable early neurologic assessment. In view of the prolonged surgery with significant blood loss, invasive arterial blood pressure monitoring is continued in the ICU. Patients with neuromuscular disease, reduced cardiorespiratory reserves, massive blood loss, or combined anterior and posterior procedures, and patients who have three-column osteotomies may need a period of ventilation to allow volume, temperature, and metabolic abnormalities to be corrected before extubation.

Fluid Management

Regardless of geographic location, and more so in undeveloped regions, careful attention must be paid to postoperative fluid management. Patients in our locality, where the air temperature and humidity are high, tend to drain for longer period of time (several days) and for this reason blood loss through the wound drain is carefully monitored and must be replaced. Decreased urine output may results from the syndrome of inappropriate antidiuretic hormone (ADH) secretion and use of hyponatremic fluids may result in hyponatremia and hypoosmolality. We alternate Ringer's lactate with dextrose saline postoperatively. A full blood count, urea, electrolytes, and creatinine as well as the coagulation profile are repeated immediately after surgery and then daily for 72 hours.

Pain Control

Good postoperative analgesia is essential to enable early mobilization and physiotherapy. We use a multimodal approach, combining a continuous infusion of morphine and acetaminophen. After 24 hours, if oral intake is tolerated, oral narcotic analgesia and acetaminophen are started and the intravenous medication is tapered down. Despite its effect on bleeding and interference with bone fusion, the nonsteroidal anti-inflammatory drug ketorolac may be added if pain control is difficult but only after 24 hours and for a period not longer than 72 hours. Some patients may require adjuvants like Lyrica (pregabalin) and/or diazepam. Essentially, analgesia is tailored to the needs of the patient. We transfer patients from the ICU to a step-down unit for 24 to 48 hours postoperative to facilitate care and close monitoring of the hemodynamic and neurologic parameters mentioned above.

▥ Chapter Summary

Dormans et al[1] and Levine[3] have addressed the tremendous health care challenges present in developing countries, which make up more than half of the world's population. Limitations such as lack of trained personnel, inadequate infrastructure, and lack of access to care are prominent in the developing world. Whereas in the developed world the most common diseases and causes of mortality have been heart and cerebrovascular diseases, in the developing world tuberculosis, the sequelae of traffic accidents, and congenital anomalies are major causes of death. Pediatric spine deformities abound in the developing world where there is little to no early intervention. Patients present late and with complex spine conditions that require expertise and sophisticated and expensive surgical treatment methods. Through a comprehensive volunteering and partnership programs with international medical device companies, FOCOS has successfully performed surgical mission programs to Ghana over a 15-year period, performing over 1,000 complex spine procedures utilizing advanced, modified, and relevant techniques for optimal outcomes. FOCOS believes in the creation of a sustainable infrastructure to provide optimal spine care[35] and to develop the treatment capability for the West Africa subregion by building a 50-bed orthopedic hospital. We have instituted a multidisciplinary team of specialists to manage complex spine deformities in pediatric patients with good outcomes. Innovations in treatment methods include comprehensive medical/surgical preoperative assessment protocols, risk stratification (FOCOS level 1 to 5), preoperative long-term halo gravity traction for severe and rigid spine deformities, implant density modifications, and aggressive postoperative management protocols.

Pearls

- One must recognize that there is very little access to specialty care in developing nations, and international volunteers must be dedicated and committed and have adequate knowledge of the resources in the developing country to develop an effective surgical treatment program.
- The Scoliosis Research Society outreach program site assessment checklist is a good guideline to follow for volunteers traveling to developing countries to set up surgical programs.
- The surgeon must be conversant with the local health problems such as malnutrition, parasitic infestation, and viral infections, as well as the need for adequate antituberculosis medication.
- Patients must be carefully selected and treatment plans well laid out for all involved including the medical, anesthesia, and nursing personnel. FOCOS level surgical risk stratification is helpful in this regard.
- In developing countries, paralysis is a recipe for disaster and early death because the environments and medical care for the paralytic are abysmal. Curve stabilization may be all that can be done safely for some patients.
- Deformity risk level downgrading with halo gravity traction can enable the surgeon to perform posterior-only surgery with posterior column osteotomy in select cases.
- If possible, intraoperative spinal monitoring should be considered, and there are international organizations willing to provide volunteer personnel and equipment. An alternative method is training the anesthesia team to do wake-up tests on demand.
- Complex procedures such as three-column osteotomies demand that the surgical team have significant experience with the procedure and adequate resources, including prolonged anesthesia, blood salvage or transfusion options, intraoperative spinal cord monitoring, and intensive care. When in doubt, stage the procedure.

Reducing implant density to reduce cost and shorten the procedure time should be considered.
- Mastering the techniques of free-hand pedicle screw placement is a must regardless of the deformity characteristics because C-arm fluoroscopy is rarely available in most operating rooms in developing countries.
- Overnight ventilator support in an ICU for complex cases and 24-hour anesthesia or intensivist coverage is highly recommended.

Pitfalls

- It is best to leave a patient alone if the treating physician or center does not have the experience and resources to treat a patient surgically.
- There is no room for surgical heroism when it comes to preserving life, and humility and admitting to not knowing what to do are good virtues. Refer patients to a well-equipped treatment center if possible.
- Volunteers traveling for short-term missions should also leave room for emergencies and give themselves at least a week or two of postoperative care.
- All the principles of universal precautions must be taken because many patients test positive for hepatitis B and C and HIV, which may not be known by the treating team.
- Intraoperative normovolemic hemodilution is a good blood salvage practice to avoid severe postoperative anemia and coagulopathy.
- Surgeons should not operate on a patient if they do not have complete information about the patient's socioeconomic status and living conditions, and about the personnel and facilities available to manage potential postoperative complications.
- Three-column osteotomies should be left for the most experienced surgical team, if possible, because of the high complication rate.

References
Five Must-Read References
1. Dormans JP, Fisher RC, Pill SG. Orthopaedics in the developing world: present and future concerns. J Am Acad Orthop Surg 2001;9:289–296
2. Fisher RC. Selected conditions common in the developing world. Instr Course Lect 2000;49:585–591
3. Levine AM. Can we make a difference? J Am Acad Orthop Surg 2001;9:279
4. Woolf AD, Pfleger B. Burden of major musculoskeletal conditions. Special Theme: Bone and Joint Decade 2000–2010. Bull World Health Org 2003;81:646–656
5. Dormans JP. Orthopaedic surgery in the developing world—can orthopaedic residents help? J Bone Joint Surg Am 2002;84-A:1086–1094
6. Murray CJL, Lopez AD. The Global Burden of Disease: A Comprehensive Assessment of Mortality and Disability From Diseases, Injuries, and Risk Factors in 1990 and Projected to 2020. Cambridge, MA: Harvard School of Public Health; 1996
7. Brotchi J. Presidential guest lecture of the 32nd annual meeting of the International Society for the Study of the Lumbar Spine: highly sophisticated neu-

rosurgery and the developing world. A permanent challenge. Spine 2006;31:1520–1521

8. Brouillette MA, Kaiser SP, Konadu P, et al. Orthopedic surgery in the developing world: workforce and operative volumes in Ghana compared to those in the United States. World J Surg 2014;38:849–857

9. Boachie-Adjei O, Yagi M, Nemani VM, et al. Incidence and risk factors for major surgical complications in patients with complex spinal deformity: a report from an SRS GOP site. Spine Deform 2015;3:57–64

10. Nemani VM, Kim HJ, Bjerke-Kroll BT, et al; FOCOS Spine Study Group. Preoperative halo-gravity traction for severe spinal deformities at an SRS-GOP site in West Africa: protocols, complications, and results. Spine 2015;40:153–161

11. Heinegård D, Lidgren L, Saxne T. Recent developments and future research in the bone and joint decade 2000–2010. Bull World Health Organ 2003; 81:686–688

12. Boachie-Adjei O, Yage M, Sacramento-Dominguez C, et al; Surgical risk stratification based on preoperative risk factors in severe pediatric spine deformity surgery. Spine Deformity Journal 2014;2:340–349

13. Boachie-Adjei O, Papadopoulos EC, Pellisé F, et al. Late treatment of tuberculosis-associated kyphosis: literature review and experience from a SRS-GOP site. Eur Spine J 2013;22(Suppl 4):641–646 Review

14. Tuberculosis into the next century. Proceedings of a symposium held on 4 February 1995 at the Liverpool School of Medicine. J Med Microbiol 1996;44:1–34

15. Rajasekaran S, Rishi Mugesh Kanna P, Shetty AP. Closing–opening wedge osteotomy for severe, rigid, thoracolumbar post-tubercular kyphosis. Eur Spine J 2011;20:343–348

16. Verma K, Lonner B, Toombs CS, et al. International utilization of the SRS-22 instrument to assess outcomes in adolescent idiopathic scoliosis: what can we learn from a medical outreach group in Ghana? J Pediatr Orthop 2014;34:503–508

17. Beals RK, Robbins JR, Rolfe B. Anomalies associated with vertebral malformations. Spine 1993;18:1329–1332

18. Kearon C, Viviani GR, Kirkley A, Killian KJ. Factors determining pulmonary function in adolescent idiopathic thoracic scoliosis. Am Rev Respir Dis 1993; 148:288–294

19. Horlocker TT, Wedel DJ. Anesthesia for orthopedic surgery. In: Barash PG, Cullen BF, Stoelting RK, eds. Clinical Anesthesia, 4th ed. Philadelphia: Lippincott Williams Wilkins; 2001:1103–1118

20. Dilger JA, Tetzlaff JE, Bell GR, Kosmorsky GS, Agnor RC, O'Hara JF Jr. Ischaemic optic neuropathy after spinal fusion. Can J Anaesth 1998;45:63–66

21. Auerbach JD, Lenke LG, Bridwell KH, et al. Major complications and comparison between 3-column osteotomy techniques in 105 consecutive spinal deformity procedures. Spine 2012;37:1198–1210

22. Mandel RJ, Brown MD, McCollough NC III, Pallares V, Varlotta R. Hypotensive anesthesia and autotransfusion in spinal surgery. Clin Orthop Relat Res 1981; 154:27–33

23. Tobias JD. Fenoldopam for controlled hypotension during spinal fusion in children and adolescents. Paediatr Anaesth 2000;10:261–266

24. Sethna NF, Zurakowski D, Brustowicz RM, Bacsik J, Sullivan LJ, Shapiro F. Tranexamic acid reduces intraoperative blood loss in pediatric patients undergoing scoliosis surgery. Anesthesiology 2005;102:727–732

25. Lonstein JE, Winter RB, Bradford DS, Ogilvie JW. Moe's Textbook of Scoliosis and Other Spinal Deformities, 3rd ed. Philadelphia: WB Saunders; 1994

26. Sacramento-Domínguez C, Yagi M, Ayamga J, et al. Apex of deformity for three-column osteotomy. Does it matter in the occurrence of complications? Spine J 2015;15:2351–2359

27. Papadopoulos EC, Boachie-Adjei O, Hess WF, et al; Foundation of Orthopedics and Complex Spine, New York, NY. Early outcomes and complications of posterior vertebral column resection. Spine J 2015;15:983–991

28. Pehrsson K, Larsson S, Oden A, Nachemson A. Long-term follow-up of patients with untreated scoliosis. A study of mortality, causes of death, and symptoms. Spine 1992;17:1091–1096

29. Akbarnia BA, Marks DS, Boachie-Adjei O, Thompson AG, Asher MA. Dual growing rod technique for the treatment of progressive early-onset scoliosis: a multicenter study. Spine 2005;30(17, Suppl):S46–S57

30. Akbarnia BA, Emans JB. Complications of growth-sparing surgery in early onset scoliosis. Spine 2010; 35:2193–2204

31. Lenke LG, Newton PO, Sucato DJ, et al. Complications after 147 consecutive vertebral column resections for severe pediatric spinal deformity: a multicenter analysis. Spine 2013;38:119–132

32. Karlin JG, Roth MK, Patil V, et al. Management of thoracic insufficiency syndrome in patients with Jarcho-Levin syndrome using VEPTRs (vertical expandable prosthetic titanium ribs). J Bone Joint Surg Am 2014;96:e181

33. Kawahara N, Tomita K, Baba H, Kobayashi T, Fujita T, Murakami H. Closing-opening wedge osteotomy to correct angular kyphotic deformity by a single posterior approach. Spine 2001;26:391–402

34. Reames DL, Smith JS, Fu KM, et al; Scoliosis Research Society Morbidity and Mortality Committee. Complications in the surgical treatment of 19,360 cases of pediatric scoliosis: a review of the Scoliosis Research Society Morbidity and Mortality database. Spine 2011;36:1484–1491

35. Scoliosis Research Society Global Outreach Site. Assessment form. www.srs.org/professionals/global-outreach-programs/forms

16

Safety and Complications in Pediatric Surgery

Stephen Lewis, Michael Dodds, and Sam Keshen

Introduction

With enhanced instruments, techniques, and skills, our ability to achieve significant corrections in severe spinal deformities has greatly improved. However, the risks to patients in terms of bleeding and neurologic injury have increased in parallel with increasingly aggressive attempts at deformity correction. Setting up a system with appropriate monitoring, careful planning of procedures, awareness of potential difficulties, and early recognition and treatment of impending problems will help create a safe environment in which manage these challenging surgeries.

A Multidisciplinary Approach to Comorbidities

Fortunately, the majority of patients undergoing spinal reconstructions are healthy children. However, the more complex deformities are often associated with congenital or syndromic conditions, and it is important to have a basic understanding of the disorders associated with the spinal deformity. A multidisciplinary approach involving pediatricians, geneticists, cardiologists, respirologists, and anesthesiologists can help ensure that the appropriate workup and plans for perioperative care are put in place.[1] Preoperative recognition of surgical risks such as latex allergies, malignant hyperthermia, sickle cell disease, and bleeding disorders can greatly reduce intraoperative stresses and facilitate a safer and more efficient flow of these complex procedures.

Malnutrition is an important preoperative consideration in pediatric surgery, and patients with severe deformities or respiratory issues are potentially at risk. Although evidence is somewhat weak, addressing the patient's nutritional status prior to surgery may minimize complications, improve wound healing, and facilitate recovery.[2]

Common conditions and their associated issues are listed in **Table 16.1**. Uncommon conditions should be studied carefully, and the available literature can help provide key insights

Table 16.1 Considerations for Common Pediatric Conditions Associated with Spinal Deformity

Syndrome	Airway/Pulmonary	Cardiovascular	Spinal	Other Considerations
Cerebral palsy	Chronic pneumonia Perioperative chest infections Reactive airway disease Aspiration	Anemia Decreased platelet count and functioning	Pelvic obliquity Pedicle morphology Osteoporosis Iatrogenic	Paralytic ileus GERD/aspiration Wound infection Pseudarthrosis Thermal homeostasis Opiate sensitivity
Neurofibromatosis	In dystrophic/severe scoliosis consider PFTs and chest CT	–	Dural ectasia Rib penetration Intraspinal neurofibromata Pedicle dysgenesis	–
Marfan's syndrome/Loeys-Dietz syndrome	Pectus excavatum Lordoscoliosis Tracheal/bronchial compression **(Fig. 16.1)**	Cardiomyopathy Aortic root dilatation Aortic aneurysms Hemorrhage	Dural ectasia Dysplastic pedicles	–
Spinal dysraphism	–	–	Deficient posterior elements Osteoporosis Hydrocephalus Shunt function	Latex and other allergy Urinary infection Wound infection Flap closure
Merosin negative muscular dystrophy: Duchenne, Becker, Merosin –ve muscular dystrophy	Restrictive lung disease	Decreased cardiac function Altered platelet function Hemorrhage loss of vascular reactivity	Steroid-induced osteoporosis	Minority have additional coagulopathies

	Pulmonary/Airway	Cardiovascular	Skeletal/Neurologic	Other
Spinomuscular atrophy	Diaphragm breathers; Difficult intubation, postoperative respiratory support	–	–	AVOID succinylcholine
Congenital muscular dystrophies	Decreased pulmonary function, postoperative infection, difficulties in extubating postoperatively	Decreased cardiac function		
Hemihypertrophy syndromes (Beckwith-Wiedemann syndrome; Proteus syndrome)		Aortic arch abnormalities; Vascular malformations; Hemorrhage		Abdominal malignancy
Skeletal dysplasias	PFTs often approach appropriate values for patient's stature		Cervical instability	
Mucopolysaccharidoses	Tracheobronchomalacia; Airway obstruction from GAG deposition; Inability to intubate/ventilate; Low airway collapse; Difficulty extubating	Coronary artery disease (later); Valve disease; Pulmonary hypertension	Cervical instability; Small pedicles; Soft bone	
Congenital scoliosis	Rib synostosis; Thoracic insufficiency	Cardiac abnormalities	Multiple anomalies; Tethering of cord diastematomyelia	VACTERL association

Abbreviations: CT, computed tomography; GAG, glycosaminoglycan; GERD, gastroesophageal reflux disease; PFT, pulmonary function test; VACTERL, vertebral defects, anal atresia, cardiac defects, tracheoesophageal fistula, renal anomalies, and limb defects.

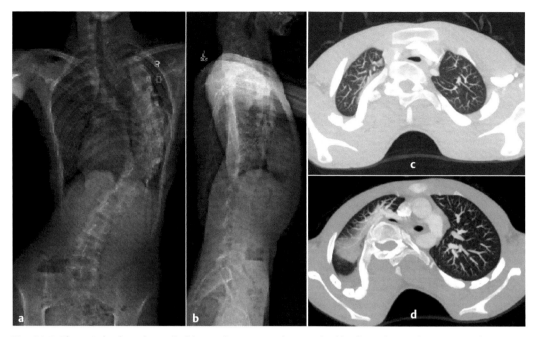

Fig. 16.1 Thoracic lordoscoliosis. **(a,b)** Standing anteroposterior (AP) and lateral radiographs demonstrate an 80-degree right thoracic curve with 25 degrees of thoracic lordosis. **(c)** Axial computed tomography (CT) confirms the anterior position of the vertebral body in the mediastinum with compression of the trachea. **(d)** Axial CT at the level of the left and right main bronchi confirms bronchial compression and right distal segmental atelectasis.

into their clinical management. For example, patients with severe fixed thoracic hyperlordosis can have mediastinal compression secondary to the spinal deformity (**Fig. 16.1**). This can lead to bronchial compression with secondary pneumonias. In these cases, extensive anterior releases followed by posterior column releases and correction can mobilize the spine sufficiently to bring the spine out of the chest to relieve this compression. Patients with neurofibromatosis frequently develop rib abnormalities with secondary migration into the spinal canal (**Fig. 16.2**), which could potentially complicate deformity correction and cause neural injury.[3] Neurofibromatosis and Marfan's syndrome are commonly associated with dural ectasia (**Fig. 16.3**). This can lead to significant difficulties in achieving fixation as well as increased incidence of dural tears and pseudarthrosis.[4] If these anatomic variations are recognized early enough, surgeons can take the time to consider alternatives such as intraoperative traction to aid in correction without fixation at every segment, and structural bone grafts to accommodate bone deficiencies.

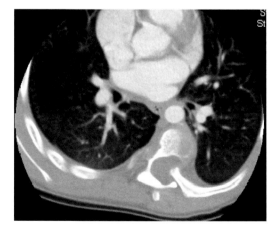

Fig. 16.2 Neurofibromatosis. Axial CT at the level of the apex of deformity demonstrates dural ectasia and rib head migration on the convexity of the curve into the spinal canal.

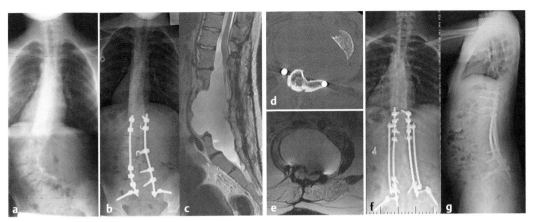

Fig. 16.3 Dural ectasia. **(a)** Preoperative AP radiograph demonstrates a dystrophic 75-degree lumbar curve in a 10-year-old girl with neurofibromatosis. **(b)** A posterior T12 to pelvis instrumentation requiring hooks and pedicle screws was used to achieve stable fixation. **(c)** Sagittal T2-weighted magnetic resonance imaging (MRI) 10 years later demonstrates progressive dural ectasia with erosion of lumbar vertebral bodies and posterior elements. **(d)** Axial CT and **(e)** MRI obtained for preoperative planning prior to revision surgery demonstrate dissociation of the anterior and posterior columns at the level of the dural ectasia. Post-revision standing long-cassette **(f)** AP and **(g)** lateral radiographs illustrate construct strengthening utilizing a bilateral double-rod technique and increased bone anchors proximally, along with structural bone graft.

Preoperative Planning

Surgical Considerations

Preoperative preparation of a case greatly improves the flow and safety of the surgical procedure. After the medical issues are addressed, the technical issues should be thoroughly reviewed. This entails ensuring that the appropriate personnel are scheduled, that the required equipment is available, and that the surgical plan with the appropriate imaging has been reviewed. Arranging an appropriate postoperative setting, such as an intensive care unit, to provide the required care and monitoring after surgery will help ensure perioperative safety and recovery.

Personnel

Surgical assistants, neuromonitoring technicians, cell saver staff, nurses, and anesthesia teams familiar with the procedure will greatly improve the flow of the surgery. Good communication between the neuromonitoring and anesthesia teams helps provide accurate and timely data on the status of the spinal cord. A nursing team familiar with the equipment and the procedure greatly improves the flow of the surgery in terms of having the appropriate instruments and implants opened and ready for use, avoiding costly delays. Capable assistants who are familiar with the surgical techniques and methods are invaluable in the efficiency and success of the procedure.

Although having an experienced team is key, the surgeon remains the captain of the ship. The surgeon should establish a positive atmosphere for the team. Good preparation provides the needed confidence that is so important in coordinating the various team members. Although the majority of cases generally run smoothly, it is when things are not going as planned that the surgeon's leadership will be most important. Remaining calm under these circumstances and coordinating with the team to ensure that the appropriate measures are taken to understand and manage the situation can help salvage difficult situations and lead to good outcomes. Warning the team ahead of time of high-risk steps in the procedure, having plans on hand for unexpected bleeding or neuromonitoring changes, and discussing the expected operative time, the desired blood pressure, and the use of antifibrinolytics with the anesthesia will help create a safe environment.

Planning a Case

"By failing to prepare, you are preparing to fail."
—Benjamin Franklin

Although some surgeons believe that there is no substitute for good intraoperative thinking, we are of the school that stresses planning as the key to success. As a case example, a 12-year-old girl presents with a large right thoracic deformity with coronal imbalance (**Figs. 16.4** and **16.5**). This case illustrates the importance of obtaining an accurate diagnosis to best plan the surgical procedure.

Clinical Presentation

The patient is a healthy 12-year-old girl. She does not take any medication and has no allergies. There is no family history of spinal deformity. She denies any cardiac, renal, or ocular issues. She has no previous surgeries. She is premenarchal. She has no café-au-lait spots and a normal neurologic examination.

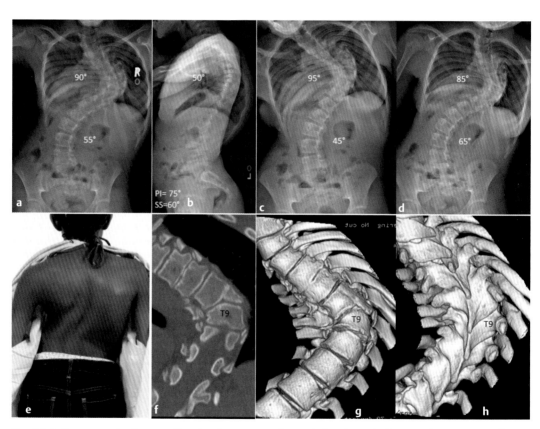

Fig. 16.4 Case example. Preoperative standing (a) AP, (b) lateral, and (c) left- and (d) right-side bending radiographs demonstrate a stiff thoracic curve. (e) Preoperative photograph demonstrates the clinical deformity with trunk shift. (f) Preoperative CT scan performed for surgical planning. Coronal slice through the apex demonstrates the partially fused right T8 hemivertebra. (g,h) Three-dimensional reconstructions show the anterior aspect of the apical deformity (g) and the posterior aspect (h) of the surgeon's view prior to posterior spinal surgery.

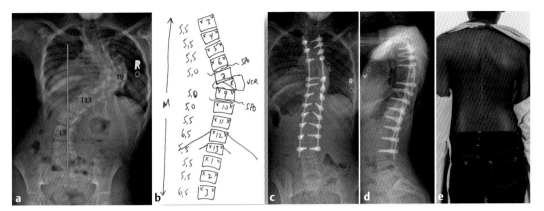

Fig. 16.5 Case example (cont'd). **(a)** Preoperative standing radiograph demonstrates rib asymmetry and trunk shift, with the center sacral vertebral line (CSVL) superimposed. **(b)** Preoperative planning "map" simplifies the key features of the deformed anatomy, the planned levels of instrumentation, the screw diameters and type, as well as the anticipated levels of osteotomies. This map is displayed in the operating room during the surgery. Postoperative standing **(c)** AP and **(d)** lateral radiographs and **(e)** clinical photograph following a T3 to L3 instrumentation with a T8 right hemivertebra resection and posterior column osteotomies at T6–T7 and T9–T10 demonstrate a well-balanced correction.

Imaging

Radiographic assessment should include the following:

- Determination of the number of thoracic and lumbar segments
- Determination of the Risser grade and the status of the triradiate cartilage
- Assessment of any coronal or sagittal deformities
- Determination of the presence of any congenital deformities
- Assessment of any spondylolisthesis
- Assessment of the pedicle size and morphology
- Assessment of any abnormal soft tissue or bony shadows
- Measurement of all curves in the coronal and sagittal planes
- Measurement of pelvic parameters (in cases involving the lumbosacral junction)

Standing radiographs in this case example demonstrate a large right thoracic curve with a secondary left lumbar curve. The patient is Risser grade 0 with closed triradiate cartilages. There are 13 ribs on the right and 12 ribs on the left. There is a small rib on the last thoracic level. There are five lumbar segments. Although the curve appears to be a large idiopathic one, closer inspection is suggestive of a congenital component. A computed tomography (CT) scan is performed showing a right-sided T8 hemivertebra, fused proximally to T7, with associated remodeling of the proximal portion of T9. A congenital fusion of T5–T6 is noted. There are 12 complete thoracic vertebrae and one hemivertebra for a total of 13 thoracic levels. Magnetic resonance imaging (MRI) (not shown) does not demonstrate any evidence of a Chiari malformation, diastematomyelia, tethered cord, or syrinx.

Preoperatve Plan

A thorough discussion is undertaken with the patient and family to determine their goals and expectations of surgical correction for the deformity. Options for correction are provided along with the expected outcomes and associated risks. In this case, the decision is made to perform a maximal correction through a posterior hemivertebra resection, supplemental periapical posterior column osteotomies, and a posterior construct. The plan is as follows:

- Instrumentation
  - A posterior instrumentation system for a 5.5-mm rod
  - An osteotomy set
  - A rod reduction system
- Anesthesia preoperative consultation
- Coordination with nurse manager for available staff and equipment
- Available intensive care unit bed
- Available neuromonitoring team
- Available cell saver technician
- Consideration of a three-dimensional (3D) printing of the CT scan to provide a model of the spine to plan the procedure and osteotomies

A surgical map (**Fig. 16.5b**) is created preoperatively with a plan for the size and location of the screws and whether the screws will be multiaxial or otherwise, the level and type of osteotomies, and the landmarks for the thoracolumbar junction. Careful analysis of the radiographs and the CT scan form the basis of this map. The nurses are able to prepare the appropriate screws allowing for greater efficiency during screw placement.

Intraoperative Procedure

The steps of the procedure should be well planned. For this case example, the steps are as follows:

1. Positioning
2. Patient preparation and draping
3. Baseline neuromonitoring
4. Exposure
5. Implant placement
6. Posterior column osteotomies
7. Hemivertebra resection
8. Osteotomy closure
9. Rod placement
10. Decortication and bone grafting
11. Wound closure

After each step, communication with the team ensures that the neuromonitoring is stable and that the blood loss is manageable with stable hemodynamics. Generally, the steps of the pro-

cedure that can entail the most blood loss are exposure, implant placement, osteotomies and decompressions, and decortication. If problems arise during any of these steps, it is important to choose the appropriate times to stop the procedure. For example, if blood loss is excessive following implant placement, the procedure can be stopped, with a second stage planned for another day.

Intraoperative "Time-Outs"

"The beginning is the most important part of the work."
—Plato, *The Republic*

When contemplating major osteotomies or vertebral column resections, obtaining good quality and sufficient anchors for stability and control is mandatory. Without these in hand, adopting a more conservative correction strategy is recommended.

Generally, we recommend a formal "time-out" prior to the major osteotomy. During this time-out, we ensure the following:

- The patient is hemodynamically stable and has acceptable reserves.
- The blood pressure is at the desired level.
- The blood loss is at an acceptable level.
- The hemoglobin is at an appropriate level.
- Blood products are available in the operating room.
- The proper equipment is available.
- The neuromonitoring is stable.
- The appropriate team members are present.
- Sufficient operating time is available.

If we are not satisfied that all these components are in place, we would elect to terminate the case at this point and stage the osteotomy for another day. If no decompression or osteotomies are performed and there is no instability, the rods would not be inserted and wound closure would be performed (**Fig. 16.6**).

It may be useful to stage a complex deformity correction so as to optimize perioperative safety. The staging should be planned if the surgeon anticipates extensive blood loss or long surgical times. In staged surgery, the procedure is generally split into exposure and implant

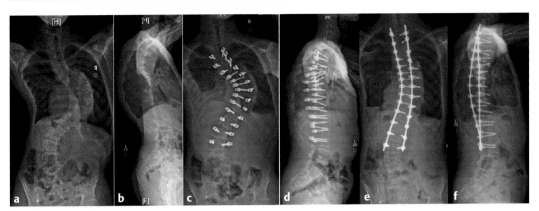

Fig. 16.6 Unplanned staged surgery. **(a,b)** Preoperative AP and **(b)** lateral radiographs of a 15-year-old boy with a rapidly progressive 95-degree right thoracic curve and suspected underlying connective tissue disorder. **(c,d)** AP and lateral radiographs following stage 1. The surgery was aborted after exposure and anchor insertion due to excessive blood loss of 2.8 L. Stage 2 was performed 6 weeks later and consisted of multiple apical posterior column osteotomies and completion of the construct from T2 to L3. **(e,f)** Postoperative AP and lateral radiograph shows the final construct.

placement on the first day, with the osteotomies and rod placement done on another day. The benefits of staging include two shorter operative days as opposed to one long day, as well as greater predictability and planning. A second stage a few days later, however, may not provide the patient with sufficient time to recover and regain sufficient nutrition. In a report by Gum et al,[5] staging was associated with greater blood loss, longer operative time, and greater length of hospital stay. Complication rates were equal in both groups. The main issues for staging are operative time and bleeding. If these can be limited, then it is more convenient for the patient and for the surgical team to proceed in one stage. Generally, we recommend good closure of the wound following the first stage in the event that, for logistical or medical reasons, the patient does not undergo the second stage in a timely manner.

Neuromonitoring

The use of multimodality neuromonitoring has greatly improved the safety of complex spinal deformity procedures by providing real-time intraoperative feedback enabling timely surgical adjustments.[6] The integrated and active participation of the neurophysiologists in the surgical team, and active communication with the surgeon and anesthesiologist cannot be overemphasized. The combination of somatosensory evoked potentials (SSEPs), motor evoked potentials (MEPs), and electromyography (EMG) provides data on the spinal cord and nerve roots. SSEP provides information related to primarily the dorsal columns. MEP provides information on the motor corticospinal tract and represents the anterior portion of the spinal cord. In this way, ischemic events involving the anterior circulation of the spinal cord cause changes in the MEP, which indirectly represent the spinothalamic tract, the other main anterior located tract.

The two main mechanisms of spinal cord injury are direct trauma and ischemia. Direct trauma to the spinal cord, through decompression, implant placement, or reduction maneuvers, can cause alerts in both the SSEP and MEP. Ischemic events related to traction, reduction, and other corrective maneuvers, will cause reduction in the MEP amplitude alone.

Vitale et al[7] have published a checklist to follow in the operating room when neuromonitoring changes occur (**Fig. 16.7**). The checklist includes gaining control of the room, reviewing the anesthetic and systemic factors, ensuring that the technical features of the monitoring

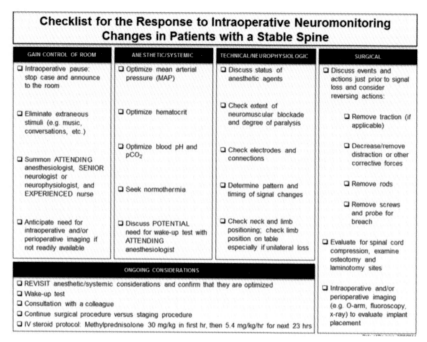

Fig. 16.7 Intraoperative neuromonitoring changes are managed according to this algorithm developed by Vitale et al. (Reproduced with permission from Vitale MG, Skaggs DL, Pace GI, et al. Best practices in intraoperative neuromonitoring in spine deformity surgery: development of an intraoperative checklist to optimize response. Spine Deform 2014;2:333–339.)

are correct, and reviewing the surgical factors that preceded the changes. Ongoing review and considerations if there is no improvement in the monitoring include performing a wake-up test, administration of steroids, consulting with a colleague, and stopping the case. Having the checklist in the room can help to provide a methodical approach to the monitoring change, with all team members aware of their roles.

When dorsally placed intra-canal implants such as hooks and sublaminar wire techniques were used, SSEP was the modality of choice as there was an increased risk of injury to the posterior part of the spinal cord. However, with pedicle screw systems and more judicious use of osteotomies, greater corrections are achieved, leading to more stretch and ischemic injuries to the spinal cord. Thus, MEP has become a much more important modality in current practice, where identifying ischemic injuries early can lead to corrective maneuvers or releases that prevent the ischemia from progressing to cord infarction and permanent motor paralysis. MEP changes are more sensitive than SSEP

recordings. In a study of intraoperative traction, all 17 cases with neuromonitoring changes demonstrated a reduction in MEP amplitude, but only one of the 17 cases demonstrated a reduction in SSEP amplitude.[8] The reduction in MEP amplitude was reversible by decreasing or removing the traction, indicative of ischemia as the basis of the change. Similarly, in a series of three-column osteotomies in children, 21 alerts were noted in 37 cases, of which all cases had MEP alerts but only three had SSEP alerts.[9] There were no cases of isolated SSEP changes. In that series, the alerts were classified based on the timing of the alerts (**Table 16.2**). Maneuvers were performed to reverse the action taken that caused the alert, leading to return of MEP signal.

It is important to note that the size of the amplitude of the MEP signal is not associated with the amount of clinical neurologic dysfunction. Any MEP signal at all suggests that spinal cord infarction has not occurred. Efforts to maintain spinal cord perfusion through hemodynamics and to maintain adequate sys-

Table 16.2 Classification of Neuromonitoring Alert Types in Three-Column Posterior Osteotomies and Actions Taken in Response to the Alerts

Alert Type	Timing	Action
1	Prior to decompression	Remove traction if present; check implants
2	During decompression	Complete decompression and close osteotomy
3	Following osteotomy closure	Open osteotomy; check for sources of compression; add or change interbody support or limit osteotomy closure and correction

Source: Jarvis JG, Strantzas S, Lipkus M, et al. Responding to neuromonitoring changes in 3-column posterior spinal osteotomies for rigid pediatric spinal deformities. Spine 2013;38:E493–E503. Reprinted by permission.

temic blood pressure and oxygen-carrying capacity are important even in the postoperative period, to protect the vulnerable spinal cord from infarcting. Although there is some controversy as to the exact level of mean arterial pressure (MAP) to maintain and for how long, maintaining the MAP at or just above the patient's baseline MAP is highly recommended. Efforts to maintain the blood pressure at too high a level may lead to unnecessary fluid overload, and the use of α-sympathetic agents that divert blood to the core organs, including the heart, kidneys, brain, and lungs, and away from the spinal cord may have a negative effect on spinal cord perfusion. Low-dose dopamine as a first-line drug followed by norepinephrine, if needed, provide more β-sympathetic activity that is preferred by the spinal cord in the setting of neurogenic shock.

The Stagnara wake-up test remains the gold standard of all monitoring.[10] With reliable MEP monitoring, it is less frequently needed. If, however, intraoperative maneuvers fail to produce the expected return of signal, it is important to have the patient and the team prepared in advance for the test so as to have a direct measure of spinal cord function. This advance preparation will help provide a more efficient and reliable test, limiting significant delays that can be associated with waking up the patient during the procedure.

Postoperative Care

The early postoperative period is very important to the success of the procedure. The immediate issues include hemodynamics, respiratory status, pain control, and neurologic function. A team capable of providing close monitoring of the vital signs and performing accurate neurologic examinations can help recognize or prevent complications such as a delayed anterior cord syndrome and ischemic cord injury, which can be associated with these cases.

Following surgery, postoperative care is centered around five main areas: (1) pain control, (2) pulmonary management, (3) gastrointestinal complications, (4) neurologic function, and (5) wound care and surgical-site infection.

Pain Control

Patient- or nurse-controlled analgesia is useful. Opiates are effective at managing early postoperative pain, although smaller aliquots are appropriate for neuromuscular patients who appear more sensitive to their side effects. Acetaminophen should be used as an adjunct to help minimize narcotic needs. Opiates should be limited to minimize respiratory and gastrointestinal complications. The use of nonsteroidal anti-inflammatory drugs is controversial because of their potential negative effects on bone healing.[11]

Pulmonary Management

Chest physiotherapy in the postoperative setting can be useful in reducing basal atelectasis. In patients with impaired pulmonary function, bi-level positive airway pressure (BiPAP) may be beneficial, and the staff should be trained in its use preoperatively. Rarer complications such as a hemothorax and chylothorax should be considered in patients that have had anterior or chest wall procedures (**Fig. 16.8**). Early

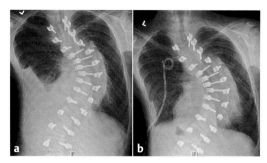

Fig. 16.8 Chylothorax after the first stage of surgery. **(a)** AP radiograph of a hydropneumothorax in the patient shown in **Fig. 16.6**. **(b)** This was managed with chest tube insertion, dietary restriction, total parenteral nutrition, and octreotide until drainage of chyle ceased. The source of the chyle leak was not determined in this case that was managed through an all-posterior approach without three-column osteotomies.

mobilization and time out of bed is likely the most important step in stimulating deep breathing and minimizing postoperative respiratory issues.

Gastrointestinal Complications

Gastrointestinal complications are frequently seen, particularly after correction of a significant deformity.[12] Paralytic ileus and superior mesenteric artery syndrome may occur, and are more difficult to identify in the uncooperative or uncommunicative pediatric patient. A 10% drop in circulating volume may be associated with a 50% decrease in gut perfusion. Patients should be placed on nil-by-mouth orders until bowel sounds are present and the patient is passing flatus. Thereafter, a gradual return to full diet is permitted. Opiate use in the postoperative period contributes to ileus, and a balance between managing pain and bowel function must be discussed with the patient and family. Less frequent complications such as Ogilvie syndrome, in which a competent ileocecal valve in combination with an ileus can cause severe dilation of the cecum with the potential for perforation, should be considered in patients with refractory ileus. In neuromuscular patients with preoperative nutritional deficiency, placement of a gastric tube

for postoperative nutrition may help to optimize postoperative nutrition and healing.

Neurologic Function

Regular spinal cord testing should be performed in the postoperative period. Postoperative hypotension and anemia may be associated with spinal cord hypoperfusion and lead to ischemic spinal cord injury. Attention to maintaining an adequate level of MAP is important, and a setting like an intensive care unit or a step-down unit may be required. It is important to ensure that the personnel with direct care of the patients, such as the nurses, residents, and house staff, are skilled in performing proper neural assessments and in recognizing and treating spinal cord syndromes. The use of medications such as steroids in the setting of spinal cord injury is controversial, with little evidence one way or the other to support its use. The preferred dose and length of treatment are at the discretion of the treating physicians.

Wound Care and Surgical-Site Infection

Surgical-site infection is one of the more important postoperative complications and the leading cause of unplanned 30-day readmission in pediatric spinal deformity surgery.[12] The rate of infections is greatest in neuromuscular scoliosis cases, with a high prevalence of mixed organisms.[13] Although some infections emanate from the inside of the wound, the majority are caused by outside bacteria tracking in.

Preventing outside-in contamination of the wounds is extremely important in preventing early postoperative infections. A tight, meticulous closure of the fascia is an extremely important component of the procedure. A subcutaneous layer closure can help protect the facial repair. Although most centers are keen on removing the Foley catheters as quickly as possible, we prefer to keep it until the patient is mobile enough to get to the bathroom or for about 3 days in nonambulatory patients. Theoretically, this practice may increase the incidence of urinary tract infections, but diverting the urine away from the wound during the critical first few days of wound healing can prevent urine contamination. The use of diapers in pediatric patients, especially neuromuscular cases with incisions extending very distally from constructs extending to the pelvis, can lead to infections with mixed organisms. The use of impervious dressings and minimizing dressing changes has been recommended as prevention for this problem.

Following a consensus review by an expert panel, Vitale et al[14] made the following recommendations to prevent postoperative wound infections:

1. If removing hair, clipping is preferred to shaving.
2. Hair removal from the operative site should be avoided.
3. Chlorhexidine-based perioperative skin preparation is preferred.
4. Vancomycin powder should be used in the bone graft and the surgical site.
5. Impervious dressings are preferred postoperatively.
6. Postoperative dressing changes should be minimized before discharge.

Spina bifida patients are at particularly high rates of postoperative infection following posterior surgery. Previous wound closures, lack of posterior musculature, and insensate skin are predisposing factors. Although posterior instrumentation in these cases is excellent for correction and stability, the lack of posterior bone is suboptimal for fusion. Because of the extremely high rate of posterior wound infections, a separate anterior fusion procedure may be performed through a separate anterior approach to achieve fusion through the levels with poor posterior bone stock. This will facilitate fusion through these levels while preventing contamination of the anterior compartment should the posterior wound become infected (**Fig. 16.9**).

Complication Rates

Even with careful planning and execution, there is still risk of surgical complications. In a review of the *Scoliosis Research Society* (SRS) database of 19,360 cases of pediatric scoliosis,[15] the overall complication rate was 10.2%, with neuromuscular patients being at highest risk, followed by the congenital and then the idiopathic etiologies. Complications include gastrointestinal disturbances, pulmonary distress, neurologic injury, and surgical-site infection (**Table 16.3**). Complication rates have been shown to be more prevalent in revision procedures, as

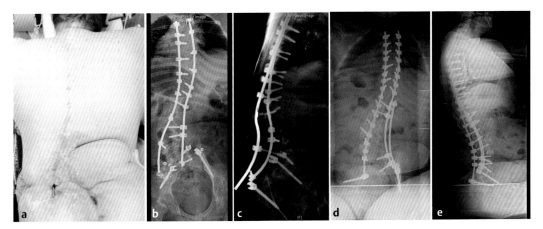

Fig. 16.9 Spinal dysraphism. **(a)** Clinical photograph of posterior instrumentation failure and deep infection following attempted posterior-only instrumented fusion 3 months following the index procedure. **(b,c)** AP and lateral radiographs demonstrate pullout of the lumbosacral fixation with posterior dislodgment of the rods. This patient was treated with wound management, revision posterior instrumentation, and a lengthy course of intravenous antibiotics. Anterior lumbar interbody fusions with tibial allografts from L1 to S1 were performed 3 months later. **(d,e)** AP and lateral radiographs 6 months post-revision shows the final construct.

Table 16.3 Complications Associated with Surgical Treatment of Scoliosis in 19,360 Pediatric Patients

Complication	Total (N = 19,360)	Idiopathic (N = 11,227)	Congenital (N = 2,012)	Neuromuscular (N = 4,657)	Other[a] (N = 1,464)
Total complications[b]	10.2% (1971)	6.3% (710)	10.6% (213)	17.9% (835)	14.5% (213)
New neurologic deficit[b]	1.0 % (199)	0.8% (86)	2.0% (41)	1.1% (49)	1.6% (23)
Death[b]	0.1% (26)	0.02% (2)	0.3% (6)	0.3% (16)	0.1% (2)
Superficial wound infection[b]	1.0% (184)	0.5% (61)	1.3% (27)	1.7% (79)	1.2% (17)
Deep wound infection[b]	1.7% (321)	0.8% (95)	0.9% (18)	3.8% (177)	2.1% (31)
Pulmonary (not embolism)[b]	1.0% (202)	0.6% (63)	1.1% (23)	1.9% (90)	1.8% (26)
Nonfatal hematologic[b]	0.5% (93)	0.2% (25)	0.1% (3)	1.2% (57)	0.5%(8)
Durotomy[b]	0.4% (76)	0.2% (22)	0.4% (8)	0.9% (42)	0.3% (4)
Implant related[b]	1.5% (296)	1.1% (120)	1.5% (31)	2.1% (100)	3.1% (45)
Deep venous thrombosis[c]	0.01% (2)	< 0.01% (1)	0.05% (1)	0% (0)	0% (0)
Pulmonary embolus[c]	0.04% (7)	0.04% (5)	0% (0)	0.0.4% (2)	0% (0)
Epidural hematoma[c]	0.02% (3)	< 0.01% (1)	0% (0)	0.02% (1)	0.1% (1)
Vision deficit[c]	< 0.01% (1)	0% (0)	0% (0)	0.02% (1)	0% (0)
Peripheral nerve/ plexus deficit[d]	0.5% (89)	0.5% (53)	0.8% (17)	0.3% (15)	0.3% (4)
SIADH[c]	0.3% (48)	0.2% (23)	0.15% (3)	0.3% (14)	0.5% (8)
Other complications[b]	2.2% (424)	1.4% (153)	1.7% (35)	4.1% (192)	3.0% (44)

Abbreviation: SIADH, syndrome of inappropriate secretion of antidiuretic hormone.
Source: Reames DL, Smith JS, Fu KM, et al; Scoliosis Research Society Morbidity and Mortality Committee. Complications in the surgical treatment of 19,360 cases of pediatric scoliosis: a review of the Scoliosis Research Society Morbidity and Mortality database. Spine 2011;36:1484–1491. Reprinted by permission.
[a] Posttraumatic, syndromic (Down, Marfan's, Ehlers-Danlos syndromes), neurofibromatosis, nonneurologic tumor, iatrogenic, bone dysplasias/dwarfism.
[b] $p < 0.001$ (Pearson p values comparing idiopathic, congenital, and neuromuscular cases).
[c] $p > 0.05$ (Pearson p values comparing idiopathic, congenital, and neuromuscular cases).
[d] $p = 0.01$ (Pearson p values comparing idiopathic, congenital, and neuromuscular cases).

well as in procedures involving anterior-only or posterior wire constructs. Complication rates have also been shown to be higher in surgeries requiring one or multiple osteotomies. Cases with osteotomies have been associated with increased blood loss, and greater risk of neurologic injury. Of the osteotomies performed, posterior column osteotomies (PCOs), Smith-Petersen osteotomies, and Ponte osteotomies present the lowest risk, whereas the three-column pedicle subtraction osteotomies and vertebral column resections have a much higher reported incidence of complications, with rates reported as high as 59%.[16] Preoperative dis-

cussions with the patient and family should explain the risks associated with these procedure, the alternative options that are available, as well as the steps that will be taken to minimize complications and correct them should they occur.

Neural Deficits

Spinal cord injury is a particularly dreaded complication of spine surgery. The rate of new neural deficit in pediatric patients is low at ~ 1%. Congenital scoliosis patients have the highest incidence of injury followed by neuromuscular patients and idiopathic patients. Of all neural injury types, incomplete spinal cord deficit is the most prevalent in pediatric deformity correction, followed by nerve root deficit and complete spinal cord deficit. Cauda equina syndrome is the least common injury type.[15] Neural complications are more prevalent in procedures involving osteotomies (2%), anterior screws only (2%), and posterior wire constructs (1.7%).

Mortality Rate

The rate of mortality in pediatric spine surgery is quite low, with a reported prevalence of only 0.1%.[17] Mortality rates in scoliotic etiologies mirror complication rates, with neuromuscular patients being most at risk, followed by congenital and idiopathic patients.[15]

⫻ Chapter Summary

The management of pediatric patients with spinal deformities is a complex process in which attention to detail and working with a knowledgeable team capable of recognizing and treating the many facets of care are imperative for good outcomes. Careful planning of cases and communication with the team can help to ensure that the required equipment and appropriate personnel are available, allowing the cases to proceed under the safest conditions while minimizing unwanted complications. Although the rate of complications is relatively low for these complex procedures, creating this safe environment can further help to decrease the frequency and severity of these unwanted events.

Pearls

- ◆ Preoperative preparation of a case greatly improves the flow and safety of the surgical procedure. This includes obtaining the appropriate imaging, conducting multidisciplinary consultations, gathering the required equipment, creating an operative plan, and ensuring that the appropriate personnel are available.

- ◆ Warning the team in advance of high-risk steps, having plans on hand for unexpected bleeding or neuromonitoring changes, and discussing the expected operative time, the desired blood pressure, and the use of antifibrinolytics with anesthesia are some of the components that create a successful environment.
- ◆ During the case, a formal "time-out" prior to performing a complex component of the procedure, such as a major osteotomy, can help ensure that the patient's hemodynamics and neuromonitoring are stable, that the blood pressure and hemoglobin are at the desired level, and that blood products and appropriate personnel are in the operating room.
- ◆ Good communication among the surgical, anesthesia, and neuromonitoring teams is essential for accurate intraoperative assessment of the patient's neurologic status. The use of a checklist in response to neuromonitoring changes can provide a systematic approach to identifying the sources of these changes.
- ◆ Postoperative care is centered around five main areas: pain control, chest management, gastrointestinal complications, neurologic function, and wound care and surgical-site infection.
- ◆ The use of chlorhexidine-based perioperative skin preparation, impervious dressings, and vancomycin powder, and minimizing dressing changes have been recommended to minimize surgical-site infections.

Pitfalls

- ◆ Patients with complex spinal deformities may have associated cardiac, respiratory, or neurologic problems that must be considered prior to surgical treatment.
- ◆ Patients with fixed hyperlordosis with bronchial compression resulting in pulmonary issues should be considered for anterior releases in association with posterior fixation to relieve the vertebral body compression of the mediastinal structures.
- ◆ Spinal deformities associated with neurofibromatosis often have associated dural ectasias along with dysplastic posterior elements. Preoperative MRI is extremely helpful in delineating this pathology.
- ◆ It is appropriate to stage a case, either planned in advance or unplanned, if the procedure is too long or because of bleeding or neuromonitoring issues. Providing sufficient time for recovery of hemodynamics and nutrition is important before performing the next stage so as to minimize complications.
- ◆ The two main mechanisms to injure a spinal cord are direct trauma and ischemia. Direct trauma to the spinal cord, through decompression, implant

◆ placement, or reduction maneuvers, can cause alerts in both the SSEP and MEP. Ischemic events related to traction, reduction, and other corrective maneuvers will cause reduction in the MEP amplitude alone.

◆ Complication rates in pediatric spinal deformity surgery are in the range of 10%. Neuromuscular and congenital scoliosis and procedures involving osteotomies have the highest rates. Fortunately, rates of mortality and neurologic complications are low.

References

Five Must-Read References

1. Blakemore LC, Perez-Grueso FJS, Cavagnaro M, Shah SA. Preoperative evaluation and decreasing errors in pediatric spine surgery. Spine Deform 2012;39–45

2. Li Y, Glotzbecker M, Hedequist D. Surgical site infection after pediatric spinal deformity surgery. Curr Rev Musculoskelet Med 2012) 5:111. doi:10.1007/s12178-012-9111-5

3. Mao S, Shi B, Wang S, et al. Migration of the penetrated rib head following deformity correction surgery without rib head excision in dystrophic scoliosis secondary to type 1 Neurofibromatosis. Eur Spine J 2015;24:1502–1509

4. Elgafy H, Peters N, Wetzel RM. Sacral erosion and insufficiency fracture secondary to dural ectasia in patient with Marfan syndrome. Spine J 2015;16: e301–302

5. Gum JL, Lenke LG, Bumpass D, et al. Does planned staging for posterior-only vertebral column resections in spinal deformity surgery increase perioperative complications? Spine Deform 2016;4:131–137

6. Thuet ED, Winscher JC, Padberg AM, et al. Validity and reliability of intraoperative monitoring in pediatric spinal deformity surgery: a 23-year experience of 3436 surgical cases. Spine 2010;35:1880–1886

7. Vitale MG, Skaggs DL, Pace GI, et al. Best practices in intraoperative neuromonitoring in spine deformity surgery: development of an intraoperative checklist to optimize response. Spine Deform 2014;2:333–339

8. Lewis SJ, Gray R, Holmes LM, et al. Neurophysiological changes in deformity correction of adolescent idiopathic scoliosis with intraoperative skull-femoral traction. Spine 2011;36:1627–1638

9. Jarvis JG, Strantzas S, Lipkus M, et al. Responding to neuromonitoring changes in 3-column posterior spinal osteotomies for rigid pediatric spinal deformities. Spine 2013;38:E493–E503

10. Thuet ED, Padberg AM, Raynor BL, et al. Increased risk of postoperative neurologic deficit for spinal surgery patients with unobtainable intraoperative evoked potential data. Spine 2005;30:2094–2103

11. Glassman SD, Rose SM, Dimar JR, Puno RM, Campbell MJ, Johnson JR. The effect of postoperative nonsteroidal anti-inflammatory drug administration on spinal fusion. Spine 1998;23:834–838

12. Martin CT, Pugely AJ, Gao Y, Weinstein SL. Causes and risk factors for 30-day unplanned readmissions after pediatric spinal deformity surgery. Spine 2015;40: 238–246

13. Croft LD, Pottinger JM, Chiang HY, Ziebold CS, Weinstein SL, Herwaldt LA. Risk factors for surgical site infections after pediatric spine operations. Spine 2015;40:E112–E119

14. Vitale MG, Riedel MD, Glotzbecker MP, et al. Building consensus: development of a Best Practice Guideline (BPG) for surgical site infection (SSI) prevention in high-risk pediatric spine surgery. J Pediatr Orthop 2013;33:471–478

15. Reames DL, Smith JS, Fu KM, et al; Scoliosis Research Society Morbidity and Mortality Committee. Complications in the surgical treatment of 19,360 cases of pediatric scoliosis: a review of the Scoliosis Research Society Morbidity and Mortality database. Spine 2011;36:1484–1491

16. Lenke LG, Newton PO, Sucato DJ, et al. Complications after 147 consecutive vertebral column resections for severe pediatric spinal deformity: a multicenter analysis. Spine 2013;38:119–132

17. Smith JS, Saulle D, Chen CJ, et al. Rates and causes of mortality associated with spine surgery based on 108,419 procedures: a review of the Scoliosis Research Society Morbidity and Mortality Database. Spine 2012;37:1975–1982

17

Measuring Outcomes in Pediatric Spinal Deformity

Sayf S.A. Faraj, Tsjitske M. Haanstra, Steven J. Kamper,
and Marinus de Kleuver

Introduction

Outcomes measurement is a fundamental component of evidence-based medicine, and it provides clinicians and patients with the information needed for shared and informed decision making. In pediatric spinal deformity care, outcome measurement has traditionally focused on the magnitude of the spinal curvature. However, in the last two decades health care systems have become more patient centered on an individual, hospital, healthcare service, and policy level. A focus on patient-centered outcome measures has implications for the daily practice of the spine surgeon as well as for patients and families, with the need for the surgeon and the family to become more actively involved in the management of the patient and the deformity. The wishes and needs of the patient require more measures than solely the radiographic ones. On a policy level, routinely measuring outcomes of care enables continuous evaluation and improvement. In the future, reimbursement may be based on value rather than on the quantity of care delivered. The transition from process measures to patient-based measures of outcome will empower surgeons and health care systems to focus on the patient's health care experience.

A basic concept in outcome measurement is the distinction between outcome domains (e.g., pain, function, walking, appearance) and the instruments that are used to measure these outcome domains (e.g., Visual Analogue Scale, Oswestry Disability Index, Spinal Appearance Questionnaire). An outcome domain can be measured with different instruments; for example, physical functioning can be measured by a "stand up and go" test or by different questionnaires about functioning. Furthermore, outcome instruments can be categorized into clinician-based outcome instruments (e.g., functional tests) and patient-reported outcome measurements (PROMs), which are questionnaires that measure perceived outcomes.

The Use of Outcome Measures

Outcome measures can be used for the following purposes: (1) treatment planning and evaluation, (2) continuous quality improvement and value-based health care, and (3) clinical research. Ideally, the same measurement instruments and measurement moments could be used for all of these purposes. Unfortunately, this is not always feasible, as each purpose requires different qualities and characteristics of a measurement instrument. For the first two purposes, it is necessary to routinely measure the outcomes in clinical practice (i.e., every patient), whereas for most research purposes a (random) sample of patients may be adequate. Routine outcome measurement is challenging, but when implemented successfully it has many benefits. For example, research has shown that asking providers to measure and report outcomes improves their performance.[1,2] Understanding and comparing outcomes facilitates continuous learning and improvement of their own strategies through learning from best practices. To make fair comparisons between institutions (so-called benchmarking), outcome measures need to be corrected for preoperative status, and risk (case mix). Comparison between observed and expected outcomes may be useful in guiding system changes for improvement of outcomes.[3]

Outcome Measurement for the Individual Patient's Treatment Planning and Evaluation

For the individual patient, outcome measures can be used in the daily practice to gain more insight into their own functioning or quality of life. They can assist in the pretreatment workup (e.g., for risk assessment) and by measuring the change between pre- and posttreatment, they help in the evaluation of the treatment. By visualizing the results, they may improve communication and help manage expectations between the caregiver and the patient. In addition, outcome measures may also be used by patients for the evaluation of individual treatment trajectories (self-management and self-monitoring). Measuring outcome for the individual patient empowers the patient to participate in informed and shared decision making regarding health care and management of spinal disorders.

Outcome Measurement for Continuous Quality Improvement and Value-Based Health Care

Outcome measures are increasingly being used for continuous quality improvement. Research has shown that asking providers to measure and report outcomes alone already improves performance.[1,2] By providing a structure for testing of changes, quality improvement methods such as plan–do–study–act (PDSA) cycles

have been used in an attempt to drive such improvements. This four-staged cyclic learning approach is aimed at the documentation of data at each stage of a treatment over time to understand natural variation in a system, increase awareness of factors that may influence outcome, and understand the impact of an intervention performance by evaluating treatment effectiveness.[4] This cycle of understanding and comparing outcome facilitates continuous learning and improvement of one's own treatment strategies through learning from best practices.

Currently in many health care systems around the world, benchmarking of outcomes and process indicators is being performed, often by stakeholders such as regulators and payers (e.g., insurance companies). In the face of these fundamental transformations in health care, it is conceivable that in the near future multiple health care systems, policymakers, governments, and payers will adjust their reimbursements based on the value (outcome per unit cost) that is created for the patient.[5] A value-based health care economy prioritizes outcome of care over volume of care, and measuring outcomes is fundamental in creating a reimbursement system that optimizes providing cost-effective care.

Outcome Measurement for Research Purposes

In research settings, outcome measures are essential in evaluating treatment effectiveness and efficacy (randomized controlled trials [RCTs], cost-effectiveness studies) and in identifying prognostic and predictive factors that may enable providers to create predictive models.

Effectiveness and Efficacy Research

In the surgical management of spinal deformities, especially in pediatrics, RCTs are challenging to conduct and are often deemed unethical. As an alternative to RCTs, observational data from routinely collected outcomes are also useful for evaluating treatment strategies.[6] It is essential to bear in mind that treatment strategies are not randomly assigned, and therefore when comparing outcomes of treatments, it is essential to try to adjust the outcomes for confounding factors, such as preoperative risk factors.

Prognosis and Prediction Modeling

Prognostic

Prognostic factors are associated with clinical outcome in the absence of treatment. These variables are helpful for defining the natural history of disease, for identifying patients at risk of contacting the disease of interest, and for determining the progression of the disease.

Predictive

Predictive factors are associated with clinical outcome following a particular treatment. These variables are helpful in identifying who will or will not benefit from a particular treatment.[7] Both prognostic and predictive factors rely on the outcome considered as an end point. Therefore, when performing research on prognostic and predictive factors for spinal deformity, it is essential to identify which outcome is being studied. For example, in cancer research, the 5-year survival rate is considered the outcome for estimating the prognosis of a particular form of cancer. For conditions such as spinal deformity, survival is not a relevant outcome. The (change in) quality of life is more relevant, which requires questionnaires evaluating the overall quality of life as an outcome for prognosis and prediction research.

Quality of Outcome Measurement/Clinimetric Properties

Measurement of patient-based health status, or patient value of a health condition, is challenging. The number of measurement instruments has increased over time, and the choice of which instrument to use has become more difficult. When choosing a measurement instrument, and this is true for questionnaires or

patient-reported measures as well as for other more objective or clinician-derived measures, it is important to take into account the quality of the instrument. The study of Terwee et al[8] features the nine most important quality criteria of outcome measures: content validity, internal consistency, criterion validity, construct validity, reproducibility, longitudinal validity, responsiveness, floor and ceiling effects, and interpretability. Depending on the design, methods, and outcomes, each criterion can be rated as negative, positive, or indeterminate. These criteria have proven to be helpful in distinguishing between low- and high-quality measurement instruments.

Which Outcomes Are Important in Pediatric Spinal Deformities?

Outcome measures in pediatric spinal deformity, which encompass the whole cycle of care, measuring overall quality of life, functioning, and disability from a patient's or caregivers perspective, will play an important role in defining appropriate care in future health care systems. The rapid growth in number and the abundant variety of measurement instruments can be confusing. Which outcome domain and instrument should be used, in light of the increasingly recognized shift toward a value-based health care from the patient's perspective?

In the evaluation of scoliosis, generic instruments, such as the Short Form Health Survey (SF-36) and the EuroQol Group Health Questionnaire (EuroQol5D), can be used to assess health-related quality of life and cost evaluations, and to compare the health status with other diseases. Currently, the only condition-specific patient-reported outcome measurements is the Scoliosis Research Society (SRS)-22 questionnaire. The SRS-22 was introduced as a condition-specific outcome measurement for adolescent idiopathic scoliosis (AIS), and it measures five outcome domains: function, pain, self-image, mental health, and satisfaction. However, outcomes domains that are measured by any instruments can differ substantially in importance for children, adolescents, and adults with spinal deformity. For example, whereas patients with adult spinal deformity (ASD) seeking reconstructive surgery mostly want relief of symptoms (e.g., pain) and improvement of quality of life, patients with AIS mostly undergo reconstructive surgery to avoid curve progression and improve self-image, rather than relief of disabling symptoms.[9] In addition to general condition-specific questionnaires such as the SRS-22, highly specific patient-reported outcome (PRO) questionnaires to assess a single outcome domain have been developed, such as the Spinal Appearance Questionnaire (SAQ) and the Trunk Appearance Perception Scale (TAPS).[10] Recently, the development of a core outcome set for adolescent deformity surgery was initiated by the Core Outcome Set for Scoliosis (COSSCO) study group (see below). As another example, using the international consensus rounds by the Nordic Spinal Deformities Society (Sweden, Denmark, Finland, Norway, and the Netherlands), a core set of 14 outcome domains (11 patient reported and 3 clinician reported) has been identified for adolescent patients with spinal deformity undergoing reconstructive surgery based on the World Health Organization's International Classification of Functioning and Disability (ICF). Clinician reported core outcome domains include "change in deformity," "complications," and "reoperation." How the remaining 11 patient reported domains out of the 14 core domains are measured by widely used patient-reported measurement instruments is presented in **Table 17.1**. Based on this analysis, a yet-to-be-defined respiratory questionnaire is needed to measure pulmonary fatigue and respiratory function.

▨ Current Developments in Outcome Measurement

Outcome measurement can only achieve its maximum benefit when the measures used are uniform, valid, and reliable. The great diversity in outcome instruments used in pediatric spinal deformity hampers the ability to compare different treatment strategies within and between care facilities, both nationally and globally.[11] It is therefore relevant for spine societies to achieve international agreement on which instrument measurements are essential to measure outcome, so that these can be implemented in future cohort studies and spine registries. To deal with this complex problem and to strive for more efficiency, the development of COSSCO was initiated. Another recent advancement in outcome measurement, relevant to many diseases and disorders including spinal deformity, is the Patient Reported Outcomes Measurement Information System (PROMIS) and the risk stratification by the Scoliosis Research Society.[12,13]

Core Outcome Set for Scoliosis

Regional and national registries have started in the Netherlands, Sweden, Finland, and the United States.[14] However, it is difficult to pool and compare outcomes between these registries because outcomes, measurement instruments, and risk stratification variables differ among those registries. Outcome registries are most valuable if they include comparable outcomes that are relevant to the patient population of interest, because this enables data pooling and benchmarking. This process will ultimately lead to improved pretreatment information on the benefits and risks of surgery for individual patients (shared decision making). Therefore, for the international community to agree on a core set of outcomes and the predictive factors (risk factors) contributing to these outcomes, the development of a core outcome set for adolescent deformity surgery for the Nordic spine registries was started. This project, supported by the AOSpine Knowledge Forum Deformity, aims to reach consensus across the Nordic Spinal Deformities Society (Sweden, Denmark, Finland, Norway, the Netherlands), about which patient-relevant outcome domains (e.g., appearance) and subsequent measurement instruments (e.g., SRS-22) are to be included in the five national spine outcome registries for adolescents and young adults (10 to 25 years of age) with a spinal deformity undergoing surgery. The development of this

Table 17.1 Core set of 11 patient reported outcome domains and subsequent measurement instruments for young patients with spinal deformity undergoing spinal surgery: Preliminary results of the COSSCO study

	Physical Function	Pain Intensity	Self-Image	Pulmonary Fatigue	Respiratory Function	Recreation and Leisure	Overall HRQOL	Satisfaction with Cosmetic Result	Physical Functioning	Pain Interference	Satisfaction with Overall Outcome
ODI	×	×							×	×	
SRS-22	×	×	×					×	×	×	×
VAS		×									
NRS		×									
SF-36	×	×				×	×		×	×	
SRS-24	×	×	×			×		×	×	×	×
SF-12	×	×				×	×		×	×	
SRS-30	×	×	×			×		×	×	×	×
JOACME	×	×		×			×		×	×	
LBOS	×	×							×	×	
RMDQ	×					×			×	×	
NDI		×				×			×	×	
SF-McGill		×								×	
DPS		×								×	
AIMS	×	×				×			×	×	
JOABPE	×	×					×		×	×	
BASDAI	×	×				×			×		
EQ-5D	×	×					×		×		
S-ESR			×								×
TAPS			×					×			
SAQ			×					×			
SGRQ				×	×						
QLPSD	×		×				×			×	×
WRVAS			×					×			
SQLI		×	×						×	×	

Source: Consensus by the Nordic Spinal Deformities Societies (Sweden, Denmark, Finland, Norway, The Netherlands).

Abbreviations: HRQOL, health-related quality of life; ODI, Oswestry Disability Index; SRS-22/24/30, Scoliosis Research Society questionnaires; VAS, Visual Analogue Scale; NRS, Numeric Rating Scale; SF-36, Short Form 36; SF-12, Short Form 12; JOACME, Japanese Orthopaedic Association Cervical Myelopathy Evaluation; LBOS, Low Back Outcome Score; RMSQ, Roland Morris Disability Questionnaire; NDI, Neck Disability Index; SF-McGill, Short Form McGill Questionnaire; DPS, Denis Pain Scale; AIMS, Arthritis Impact Measurement Scale; JOABPE, Japanese Orthopaedic Association Back Pain Evaluation Questionnaire; BASDAI, Bath Ankylosing Spondylolitis Disease Activity Index; EQ-5D, EuroQol 5D; S-ESR, Self-Esteem Scale by Rosenberg; TPAS, Trunk Appearance Perception Scale; SAQ, Spinal Appearance Questionnaire; SGRQ, St. George's Respiratory Questionnaire; QLSPD, Quality of Life Profile for Spine Deformities; WRVAS, Walter Reed Visual Assessment Scale; SQLI, Scoliosis Quality of Life Index.

AOSpine core outcome set for young adolescents and adults undergoing reconstructive spinal surgery will be implemented in the five national spine outcome registries, and this will facilitate comparisons across studies, registries, and nations to improve the quality of daily clinical practice. A core outcome set for patients with adult spinal deformity and neuromuscular spinal deformity is also being developed.

PROMIS and Computer-Adaptive Testing

The Patient Reported Outcomes Measurement Information System (PROMIS) aims to be a system of reliable, precise measures of patient–reported health status for physical, mental, and social well–being funded by the United States National Institutes of Health (NIH). PROMIS is currently being validated and calibrated in many patient groups throughout the United States and Europe, although not yet in populations undergoing surgery for spinal deformities. PROMIS scales, once validated for a specific patient group, may be calibrated and built into computer adaptive tests that integrate the advances in measurement theory and the power of computer technology to administer a PRO instrument that selects questions on the basis of a patient's response to previously administered questions (or possibly other prior information). Highly informative questions are selected so that we may estimate scores that represent a person's standing on a domain (e.g., physical functioning, depression) with the minimal number of questions without a loss in measurement precision.[12]

Scoliosis Research Society: Risk Stratification Task Force

Identifying pretreatment risk factors for an outcome will enable gathering better patient information (shared decision making on which treatment is optimal for the individual patient) and will enable fairer comparisons and benchmarking between institutions and health care providers (by correction for patient and surgery complexity). For pediatric spinal deformity, multicenter, regional, and national registries have started to measure outcomes and to evaluate the effectiveness of treatment.[14] But it is still difficult to pool and compare outcomes between these registries because outcome domains, measurement instruments, and risk stratification variables differ. This leads to wasted opportunities to improve techniques and service delivery, as well as to poor understanding of treatment effectiveness. Before fair comparisons can be made, correction for patient risk factors such as body mass index (BMI), comorbidities, and smoking history (i.e., risk stratification) is required. Risk stratification is the use of evidence to assist in predicting (unfavorable) outcomes and complications. To achieve adequate adjustment for risk (risk stratification) in pediatric spinal deformity surgery, it is essential to commit to measuring a minimum sufficient set of pretreatment risk factors and outcome domains by using the same measurement instruments with well-defined methods for their collection and risk adjustment.

▥ Chapter Summary

Outcome measures in pediatric spinal deformity that encompass the whole cycle of care, measuring overall quality of life, functioning, and disability from a patient's or caregiver's perspective, will play an important role in future health care systems that prioritize value-based care. In the evaluation of health status, outcome instruments may have generic (e.g., overall quality of life), condition-specific (e.g., back pain), or highly specific (e.g., AIS appearance) features. Using a standard core set of instruments that measure the most relevant outcome domains and risk stratification variables for patients with spinal deformity is necessary to enable pooling and comparison of clinical outcomes, and to guide an evidence-based approach to appropriate care for patients with spinal deformity.

◆ There is a global shift toward value-based health care, which confronts all clinicians with the need to measure the value and outcome of their treatment.

◆ Outcome measures can be used for the individual patient's treatment evaluation, continuous quality improvement, value-based health care, and research purposes.

◆ Measurement instruments from a patient's perspective are recommended to directly measure the patient's health care experience.

◆ Outcome instruments may have generic (e.g., overall quality of life), condition-specific (e.g., back pain), or highly specific (e.g., AIS appearance) features.

◆ International agreement on outcome domains, measurement instruments, and risk stratification variables is essential to pool and compare clinical outcome among institutions, and to guide an evidence-based approach to care.

◆ Process measures alone (e.g., radiographic measures, complications) have a poor correlation with patients' perception of their health care experience and satisfaction with care.

◆ Implementation of measurement instruments that are not uniform, valid, and reliable to evaluate clinical outcome in pediatric spinal deformity should be avoided.

◆ Comparison of outcomes of care without risk stratification may lead to inappropriate recommendations regarding appropriate and optimal care.

References

Five Must-Read References

1. Parsons HM. What happened at Hawthorne?: New evidence suggests the Hawthorne effect resulted from operant reinforcement contingencies. Science 1974;183:922–932

2. Porter ME. What is value in health care? N Engl J Med 2010;363:2477–2481

3. Spence RT, Mueller JL, Chang DC. A novel approach to global benchmarking of risk-adjusted surgical outcomes: beyond perioperative mortality rate. JAMA Surg 2016;151:501–502

4. Taylor MJ, McNicholas C, Nicolay C, Darzi A, Bell D, Reed JE. Systematic review of the application of the plan-do-study-act method to improve quality in healthcare. BMJ Qual Saf 2014;23:290–298

5. Porter ME. A strategy for health care reform—toward a value-based system. N Engl J Med 2009;361:109–112

6. Weinstein JN, Lurie JD, Tosteson TD, et al. Surgical compared with nonoperative treatment for lumbar degenerative spondylolisthesis. four-year results in the Spine Patient Outcomes Research Trial (SPORT) randomized and observational cohorts. J Bone Joint Surg Am 2009;91:1295–1304

7. Italiano A. Prognostic or predictive? It's time to get back to definitions! J Clin Oncol 2011;29:4718, author reply 4718–4719

8. Terwee CB, Bot SDM, de Boer MR, et al. Quality criteria were proposed for measurement properties of health status questionnaires. J Clin Epidemiol 2007; 60:34–42

9. Bridwell KH, Shufflebarger HL, Lenke LG, Lowe TG, Betz RR, Bassett GS. Parents' and patients' preferences and concerns in idiopathic adolescent scoliosis: a cross-sectional preoperative analysis. Spine 2000;25:2392–2399

10. Bagó J, Climent JM, Pérez-Grueso FJS, Pellisé F. Outcome instruments to assess scoliosis surgery. Eur Spine J 2013;22(Suppl 2):S195–S202

11. Porter ME, Larsson S, Lee TH. Standardizing patient outcomes measurement. N Engl J Med 2016;374: 504–506

12. Cella D, Yount S, Rothrock N, et al; PROMIS Cooperative Group. The Patient-Reported Outcomes Measurement Information System (PROMIS): progress of an NIH Roadmap cooperative group during its first two years. Med Care 2007;45(5, Suppl 1)S3–S11

13. Wang K, Vitale M. Risk stratification: perspectives of the patient, surgeon, and health system. Spine Deform 2016;4:1–2

14. van Hooff ML, Jacobs WCH, Willems PC, et al. Evidence and practice in spine registries. Acta Orthop 2015;86:534–544

Index